Preventing Youth Problems

Issues in Children's and Families' Lives

Series Editors:
Thomas P. Gullotta, *Child and Family Agency of Southeastern Connecticut, New London, Connecticut*
Herbert J. Walberg, *University of Illinois at Chicago, Chicago, Illinois*
Roger P. Weisberg, *University of Illinois at Chicago, Chicago, Illinois*

PREVENTING YOUTH PROBLEMS
Edited by Anthony Biglan, Margaret C. Wang, and Herbert J. Walberg

A Continuation Order Plan is available for this series. A continuation order will bring delivery of each new volume immediately upon publication. Volumes are billed only upon actual shipment. For further information please contact the publisher.

Preventing Youth Problems

Edited by

Anthony Biglan

Oregon Research Institute
Eugene, Oregon

Margaret C. Wang

Temple University
Philadelphia, Pennsylvania

and

Herbert J. Walberg

University of Illinois at Chicago
Chicago, Illinois

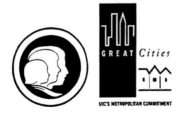

Kluwer Academic / Plenum Publishers
New York • Boston • Dordrecht • London • Moscow

Library of Congress Cataloging-in-Publication Data

Preventing youth problems/edited by Anthony Biglan, Margaret C. Wang, and Herbert
J. Walberg.
     p.   cm. — (Issues in children's and families' lives)
  Includes bibliographical references and index.
  ISBN 0-306-47733-5
     1. Child development.   2. Child psychology.   3. Clinical child psychology.   4. Adolescent
psychology.   I. Biglan, Anthony.   II. Wang, Margaret C.   Walberg, Herbert J., 1937–
IV. Issues in children's and families' lives (Kluwer Academic/Plenum Publishers)

HQ772.P74 2003
305.231—dc21
                                                                              2003044645

ISBN: 0-306-47733-5

©2003 Kluwer Academic / Plenum Publishers, New York
233 Spring Street, New York, New York 10013

http://www.wkap.nl

10 9 8 7 6 5 4 3 2 1

A C.I.P. record for this book is available from the Library of Congress

Permissions for books published in Europe: *permissions@wkap.nl*
Permissions for books published in the United States of America: *permissions@wkap.com*

Printed in the United States of America

Acknowledgments

As series editors, we greatly appreciate Anthony Biglan for first envisioning the project for this book and the late Margaret Wang for enthusiastically joining the work and making it happen. They recruited a distinguished group of scholars who brought their insights and evidence to bear upon the important topic of this volume—the prevention of important youth behavior problems. The chapter authors identify recent trends and make recommendations for the best means of preventing behavioral problems among today's youth.

Both the national invitational conference and the book chapters were sponsored by the Laboratory for Student Success, the Mid-Atlantic regional educational laboratory, at Temple University Center for Research in Human Development and Education (TUCRHDE) through a contract with the Office of Educational Research and Improvement (OERI) of the U.S. Department of Education. Some of the work on this book was also supported by the Center for Advanced Study in the Behavioral Sciences through funding provided by the Robert Wood Johnson Foundation (grant # 034 248) and the National Science Foundation (grant # BCS 960 1236), as well as grants from the National Institute on Drug Abuse (DA 12202) and the National Cancer Institute (CA86169 and CA38273).

At the invitational conference, the chapter authors benefited from discussions with one another, other scholars, policy makers, educators, and parents. Their recommendations are reported in the last chapter. Under Margaret Wang's leadership of the Laboratory, Julia St. George and Marilyn Murphy helped plan and coordinate the conference to ensure it was well managed and productive. Lydia Hoag provided splendid editorial service in preparing the manuscript for publication. In addition, Christine Cody of the Oregon Research Institute worked tirelessly on aligning references, proofreading, and assisting with the copyediting of the manuscript.

Margaret C. Wang provided much of the energy that made this project and volume possible. Her untimely passing shocked many scholars and educators. They were unaware of the battle she waged so valiantly against her disease even as the conferences and editing took place. Her spirit will continue to inspire and guide us and others.

HERBERT J. WALBERG
ROGER WEISSBERG
Series Editor

Contents

Introduction

Anthony Biglan and Herbert J. Walberg

This book provides information needed to prevent five of the most common, costly, and dangerous problems of adolescence: anti-social behavior, tobacco use, alcohol and drug abuse, and sexual behavior that risks disease and unwanted pregnancy. Over the past 30 years, scientific research on children and adolescents identified the major conditions influencing each of these problems. The research provides information for designing programs and policies that prevent such problems. We hope that compiling this information in a single volume will foster better use of research findings.

Adolescent Problem Behaviors

Preventing the problems discussed in this volume would be of substantial benefit to many young people and to society as a whole. Consider tobacco use. Each year about 400,000 people die in this country as a result of smoking-related illnesses. Most smoking begins in adolescence (U.S. Department of Health and Human Services, 1994). Of the nearly 3,000 young people who begin smoking each day, about 1,000 will die prematurely due to a smoking-related illness (Gilpin, Choi, Berry, & Pierce, 1999). Clearly, preventing young people from smoking provides substantial benefits to the health of the nation.

A similar case can be made for preventing each of the other problems addressed in this book. Antisocial behavior includes murder, aggravated assault, sexual assault, gang fights, car theft, theft of something worth more than $50, breaking and entering, strong-arming someone (Elliot, Huizinga,

& Menard, 1989). The percentage of young people accounting for these crimes ranges from 12% for murder up to 30% for robbery (Snyder & Sickmund, 1999). Alcohol abuse contributes to alcohol-related car crashes, one of the leading killers of teenagers. Among eighth graders, 15% reported binge drinking in the past two weeks, while 31% of 12th graders reported such binging. Nine percent of eighth graders and 33% of 12th graders reported being drunk in the past 30 days (Johnston, O'Malley, & Bachman, 1999). Drug abuse contributes to HIV/AIDS infections, viral and bacterial infections, and is associated with numerous psychiatric disorders. Maternal drug abuse contributes to problems in fetal development and child neglect after birth (Institute of Medicine, 1996). Sexual behavior that risks pregnancy and sexually transmitted disease results in about 25% of teens getting a sexually transmitted disease. In addition to AIDS, young people are contracting a variety of sexually transmitted diseases that contribute to cervical cancer and infertility (Landry, Singh, & Darroch, 2000). Seventy-eight percent of teen pregnancies are unplanned (Landry et al., 2000) and teenage childbearing is associated with greater risk of behavioral and academic difficulties in children. The prevention of these problems could prevent many premature deaths and much disability and would enrich the lives of many people.

The Organization of This Volume

Each of the following five chapters provides a concise summary of what is known about one of these problem behaviors. Each begins with a summary of what is known about the incidence, prevalence, and cost of the problem. This information is vital for gauging the importance of preventing the problem and for making the case for such efforts in public discussion of our priorities.

The chapters then summarize what is known about the biological and environmental influences that increase or decrease the likelihood of these problems. Those engaged in youth policy and practice need to know both the causes and solutions of these problems if they are to design the best programs for prevention, recovery, and remedy. As the chapters show, much is known about how biological conditions interact with family, peer, school, and community influences to make problems more or less likely. They also show that to a great extent all of these problems stem from the same set of home, school, peer, and neighborhood conditions—a fact that is of great importance for developing efficient preventive methods. There are, however, some conditions, such as ready access to alcohol, that uniquely influence any single behavior, and these factors cannot be ignored.

Each chapter then describes principles, programs, and policies that have been shown to reduce the incidence of each problem. For each problem, a wealth of evidence is summarized on how problem causes can be modified. Using this information can enable us to prevent adolescent problems. We hope that such information will prove useful in the United States and the rest of the world.

The next-to-last chapter identifies generic strategies for youth development prevention identified in the preceding chapters. Prevention strategies typically involve one or more of seven features. These strategies tend to improve the physical well-being of adolescents. They make use of high levels of positive reinforcement of skilled and prosocial behavior of young people. They minimize opportunities to practice behavior that will get them into trouble. They provide consistent *but mild* negative consequences for undesirable behavior.

These strategies work best when responsible adults monitor adolescents' activities. They need to reinforce desirable behavior, guide them away from situations that increase problem behavior, and ensure that problem behavior is discouraged. They provide models of desirable behavior through vicarious experiences and living examples. They teach young people, using the most effective instructional practices. These features of effective programs may be thought of as the building blocks for effective childrearing in homes, schools, and communities.

As explained in the Acknowledgments, questions and implications of the pre-circulated draft chapters in this book were intensely discussed by the authors, other scholars, educators, and youth workers in small groups. Rather than reviewing again the chapter findings, the participants concentrated on the next-step recommendations derived from the chapters, related scholarship, and their own practical and policy experiences. Their recommendations are synthesized in the final chapter of this book.

References

Elliot, D.S., Huizinga, D., & Menard, S. (1989). *Multiple problem youth: Delinquency, substance use and mental health problems.* New York: Springer-Verlag.

Gilpin, E.A., Choi, W.S., Berry, C.C., & Pierce, J.P. (1999). How many adolescents start smoking each day in the United States? *Journal of Adolescent Health, 25,* 248–255.

Institute of Medicine (1996). *Pathways of addiction: Opportunities in drug abuse research.* Washington, D.C.: National Academy Press.

Johnston, L.D., O'Malley, P.M., & Bachman, J.G. (1999). *National survey results on drug use from the Monitoring the Future study, 1975–1998 Volume I: Secondary school students,* NIH Pub. #99-4660. Rockville, MD: National Institute on Drug Abuse.

Landry, D.J., Singh, S., & Darroch, J.E. (2000). Sexuality education in fifth and sixth grades in U.S. public schools, 1999. *Family Planning Perspectives, 32(5),* 212–9

Snyder, H.N., & Sickmund, M. (1999). *Juvenile offenders & victims: 1999 National Report* (Rep. #NCJ 178257). Washington, DC: Office of Juvenile Justice & Delinquency Prevention.
U.S. Department of Health and Human Services. (1994). *Preventing tobacco use among young people: A report of the Surgeon General.* Atlanta, Georgia: USDHHS, Public Health Service, Centers for Disease Control and Prevention, National Center for Chronic Disease Prevention and Health Promotion, Office on Smoking and Health.

Chapter 1

The Prevention of Antisocial Behavior

Beyond Efficacy and Effectiveness

Philip A. Fisher

Every year in the United States, millions of dollars and countless hours of mental health, school, law enforcement, and medical personnel time are devoted to addressing antisocial child behavior in the context of families, schools, and community settings. Such efforts indicate the epidemic nature of antisocial behavior in this country. One needs only to turn to statistics concerning youth violence and criminal behavior in the United States to understand the magnitude of the problem. For example, compared to other industrialized countries, the U.S. homicide rate in 15- to 24-year-old males is more than four times that of the runner-up, with about one half of arrests in that age group involving juveniles under the age of 21 (Fingerhut & Kleinman, 1990; World Health Organization, 1992). Over the last decade in the U.S., the rate of homicides by younger adolescents has increased (Greenwood, Model, Rydell, & Chiesa, 1996). Youth are victims of violent crime at a rate that is nearly three times higher than the rate for adults (Sickmund, Snyder, & Poe-Yamagata, 1997), and youth are most frequently the perpetrators of crimes against other youth (Snyder & Sickmund, 1995).

Incidence rates for less extreme forms of antisocial behavior, such as physical fighting, stealing, and non-compliance, are also cause for concern. Such behaviors have long been the most frequent reason that children are referred to mental health clinics. Children with disruptive behavior account for almost one half of all referrals (Robins, 1981; Wolff, 1961). Roughly 2% of girls and 7% of boys meet the criteria for a disruptive behavior disorder during elementary school (Offord, Boyle, & Racine, 1991), 2%–10% of girls and 3%–16 % of boys meet the criteria during middle school (Cohen, 1993; McGee, Feehan, Williams, & Anderson, 1992), and 4%–15% of boys and girls meet the criteria during high school (Cohen, 1993; Offord et al., 1991). Thus, using even the most conservative estimates, from 1 to 4 million children and adolescents currently exhibit a disruptive behavior disorder in this country. Moreover, when treatment and other forms of intervention fail, the sequelae of child antisocial behavior are evident in the growing prison population, in the number of uneducated and unemployed individuals dependent on public assistance, in the increasing number of children in the child welfare system because of abuse and neglect, and in the overcrowded homeless shelters and substance abuse treatment programs nationwide.

This is not to argue that antisocial behavior is the single cause of these ills or that a troubled childhood guarantees problems later in development. However, decades of longitudinal research have provided strong evidence that antisocial behavior is stable across time—from a probabilistic perspective, antisocial behavior follows an identifiable trajectory from childhood, through adolescence, and into adulthood (Farrington, 1995; Loeber, 1982; Moffitt, 1993; Olweus, 1979; Patterson, DeBaryshe, & Ramsey, 1989; Patterson, Reid, & Dishion, 1992; Reid & Eddy, 1997). Parenting processes and other factors that are related to children becoming oppositional and defiant in early childhood are highly predictive of academic failure and peer rejection in primary school (Moffitt, 1993; Patterson, Capaldi, & Bank, 1991); these are in turn strongly connected to early substance use, association with delinquent peers, and other high risk behaviors (Dishion, French, & Patterson, 1995). Troubled adolescents are also more likely to become dysfunctional adults with higher rates of incarceration, troubled and failed marriages, and other problems (Reid, 1993).

Although this suggests a rather pessimistic outlook, it has at least one positive aspect. The increased understanding about the development of antisocial behavior provides clear targets for intervention and prevention. Recent research has shown that, although antisocial behavior may appear intractable in the face of traditional psychotherapeutic methods, it can be prevented and can often be treated effectively after it has developed; however, as we will see, interventions must cut across ecological systems in order to have a chance of succeeding (Borduin et al., 1995; Chamberlain & Reid, 1998; Hogue & Liddle, 1999; Reid & Eddy, 1997).

This paper provides a conceptual framework for understanding how antisocial behavior emerges in childhood. This framework helps to clarify why particular prevention and intervention programs have succeeded while other treatment approaches have failed. Age-specific programs with the strongest evidence of effectiveness are also reviewed. In addition, issues are discussed that have arisen when researcher-developed interventions have been disseminated into communities. Finally, we present a decision-making model regarding the balance between researcher-initiated and community-initiated prevention efforts in the development of future research initiatives.

The Development of Antisocial Behavior: Current Knowledge and Theoretical Confluence

A number of theories have been advanced to account for the development of antisocial behavior. Shaw, Bell, and Gilliom (2000) described the evolution of theoretical perspectives in this area, citing such early work as Hirschi's (1969) social control theory. In the 1980s, Patterson's (1982) seminal work describing the development of coercive family interaction patterns from a behavioral perspective emerged as a dominant theory of antisocial behavior. Perspectives from attachment theory (e.g., Sroufe, 1983) and social information processing (e.g., Dodge, Pettit, Bates, & Valente, 1995; Dodge & Schwartz, 1997) have been proposed more recently by researchers who question the adequacy of behavioral phenomena in accounting for the full spectrum of antisocial behavior disorders. In the 1990s, a debate emerged between behavior geneticists and researchers working from other perspectives regarding whether antisocial traits represent a stable, unalterable predisposition or whether personality is malleable and is dependent on experience (Cadoret, Yates, Throughton, Woodworth, & Stewart, 1995; DiLalla & Gottesman, 1989; Gottesman & Goldsmith, 1994; Neiderhiser, Reiss, & Hetherington, 1996; Plomin, Nitz, & Rowe, 1990).

While these various emphases might convey a sense that the field is splintered, there are also efforts to move towards consolidation. A number of researchers have embraced pragmatic approaches that incorporate disparate theoretical concepts and that emphasize theoretical confluence. Greenberg, Kusche, and Speltz (1991), for example, proposed an "ABCD Model," which incorporated cognitive, affective, behavioral, and dynamic components. Shaw et al. (2000) proposed an "early starter model" of antisocial behavior, incorporating concepts from attachment theory, social cognition theory, and coercion theory. Moreover, in a recent paper, Patterson and Fisher (2002) argue that the adequacy of any particular explanation for the development of antisocial behavior should be evaluated in terms of (a) the parsimony of that explanation (i.e., are the phenomena accounted for in the simplest and most straightforward manner possible?), (b) whether correlational evidence can be obtained that links antisocial behavior with

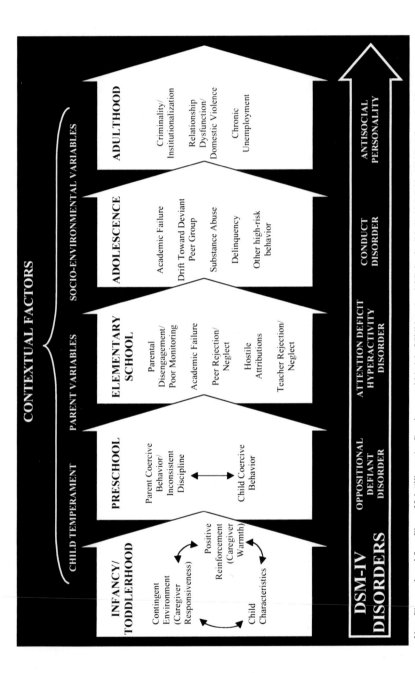

Figure 1. A model for the development of antisocial behavior.

Note. Figure adapted from Figure 32.1, "Illustrative Developmental Model of Child Antisocial Behavior," in Reid & Eddy (1997). Adapted with permission of the author.

its hypothetical causes of the development, and (c) whether experimental manipulations of the supposed causes impact any relevant outcomes. With these guidelines in mind, the following integrative perspective on the development of antisocial behavior is offered (see Figure 1), which emerges largely from a social learning tradition, but—as with Shaw et al. (2000)—it also incorporates concepts from attachment and social cognitive theory.

At the center of this model is the idea that healthy development is dependent on the early establishment of two conditions between infant and caregiver: (1) clear and predictable contingencies and (2) high levels of positive reinforcement. These concepts have conceptual overlap with constructs central to attachment theory. In particular, the establishment of contingencies is commonly referred to under the rubric of maternal sensitivity (Ainsworth, Bell, & Stayton, 1971, 1972; Kochanska, 1998; Smith & Pederson, 1988). Sensitive caregivers are described as able to identify and interpret the cues of an infant and able to respond to such cues quickly, thus meeting the infant's needs. Similarly, there is a connection between the attachment theory concept of maternal warmth (Kochanska, 1997, 1998) and the notion of high rates of positive reinforcement, especially when reinforcement is framed in terms of verbal and nonverbal encouragement on the part of the caregiver. Because of the overlap in these concepts, it is less necessary to argue in favor of one theoretical perspective over another. Rather, it may be argued that different terminology has been used to describe highly similar phenomena and that there is greater theoretical consensus than has been previously acknowledged.

Returning to the model, to the extent that the circumstances described above characterize the early environment, typical developmental processes are predisposed to occur. However, factors within the child, the parent, or the larger social context may interfere with these processes. For instance, children may be temperamentally difficult to manage, parents may fail to recognize when a child is attempting to initiate an interaction or may be predisposed to respond in a negative manner toward the child, or the family may live under highly stressful conditions (thus, parents may be distracted from attending to the needs of the child). Under any of these circumstances, caregivers may fail to respond in a consistent manner, thereby interfering with the development of clear contingencies. They may also resort to more power assertive, affectively negative behaviors to terminate distress on the part of the infant. Over time, this could lead to interactional patterns between caregiver and child in which unpleasant exchanges are terminated by high-intensity negative behavior by the parent or child. These "escape contingencies" would be expected to increase in magnitude over time.

By toddlerhood, children who have been exposed to these processes are at risk for noncompliant and coercive behavior. As they enter the social realm outside their family, they are predisposed to be rejected in interactions with peers and to be perceived as problematic by adults outside of the family—teachers in particular. According to Shaw et al. (2000), the lack of contingent responses by caregivers results in a failure to develop a sense of trust, which, in combination with frequent coercive interactions with caregivers, results in perceptions that the world is an unfriendly, unsafe place. Consequently, there may be a greater tendency for these children to attribute negative motives and other the hostile attributions towards others, as described in social cognition theory (Dodge & Schwartz, 1997).

Research on the antisocial trajectory by Patterson and colleagues (Patterson, 1982; Patterson et al., 1992; Reid & Patterson, 1989) has documented that children with high rates of noncompliant, oppositional behavior typically struggle with the transition to primary school. In particular, they are perceived by teachers as more problematic and are typically less liked by their peers. In addition, they commonly experience difficulty meeting the behavioral and academic expectations of the primary school classroom. Over the course of the primary school years, as negative behavior in the family context escalates and as children experience multiple failures in academic and social domains at school, children become increasingly alienated from the mainstream academic and social environment.

In middle school, there is a tendency for such children to associate with other rejected peers. By this time, the parents of these children are more likely to be disengaged from the parenting process owing to aversive interactions with their children. As a result, their children are poorly monitored about their comings and goings in the community and about the extent to which their peer group provides positive or negative social experiences.

Often, as such children enter high school, they increasingly associate with a rejected, deviant peer group. They are at risk for poor school attendance, for continuing academic failure, for high school dropout, and for high rates of substance use and delinquent behavior. In addition, these youth are at high risk for precocious sexual behavior and other high-risk activities. Following these trajectories into adulthood, one commonly finds high rates of chronic unemployment, dysfunctional relationships, multiple marriages, children born out of wedlock, and incarceration (Patterson et al., 1992).

In addition to this early starter model of the development of antisocial behavior, other research has documented that some children enter the antisocial trajectory at a later age (commonly early- to mid-adolescence). Late entry into this trajectory is frequently precipitated by transitions and other disruptive events in the environment of the child, including parental divorce, family relocation, and various forms of psychological trauma to the individual. In contrast to early starters, "late starters" typically appear less likely to maintain stable antisocial behavior through adolescence and into adulthood (Patterson, 1982; Patterson et al. 1992; Shaw et al., 2000).

Prevention Science Confronts Antisocial Behavior

Having described a model for the development of antisocial behavior, we now consider the methodological framework within which prevention research on antisocial behavior has been conducted. Research to date reflects the intractability of antisocial behavior in the face of traditional psychotherapeutic methods. It tends to exercise maximal control in the development, implementation, and evaluation of programs, and in its application of high levels of intervention dosage to research participants (e.g. numerous contacts or treatment sessions with families over periods of one year or more and multi-component intervention packages that included work with children and parents across several contexts). Randomized efficacy trials have emerged as the standard for evaluating prevention interventions. Within this approach, individuals are randomly assigned at the participant level or at the group level (e.g., classroom, school, or community) to experimental or control conditions. Both groups are followed across time to determine whether the intervention has impacted relevant outcome variables. To further maximize the degree of control in the investigation, researchers frequently hire and train their own staff and deliver services in highly specialized settings and service delivery programs that often do not exist in community settings. The goal of efficacy trials is to determine whether, under the best circumstances, the intervention is likely to have an impact. If an intervention shows a positive impact on important outcomes in the efficacy trials, the intervention model is then disseminated into community settings and is further evaluated in effectiveness trials.

Many positive results have emerged from research that has followed this "efficacy-to-effectiveness" approach. In the section that follows, we review the literature using a framework that places prior research along a number of different continua, which include age (infancy through adolescence), context (individual, family, extra-familial caregivers [e.g., foster parents], school, and community), severity of pathology (universal, indicated, or selected), and socioeconomic/cultural diversity.

Empirical Evidence that Antisocial Behavior Can be Prevented

Extensive literature documents outcomes from antisocial behavior prevention programs. The goal of this paper is not to provide an exhaustive review of all programs having empirical support. Rather, the review that follows provides exemplars of preventive interventions that fall at various places along the continua, using age of the child as the central organizing factor.

Prenatal and Childhood Interventions

Evidence of the intergenerational transmission of antisocial behavior (e.g., Farrington, 1995) has led to the development of interventions that are targeted at high-risk populations prior to the actual development of antisocial behavior. These interventions focus on reduction of risk factors during pregnancy and shortly after childbirth. The work of Olds and colleagues has been especially influential in this area (Olds, Henderson, Tatelbaum, & Chamberlin, 1988; Olds & Korfmacher, 1997). Olds developed a program involving home visitation with high-risk families. The project utilized a randomized trial design within which data have been gathered from a longitudinal sample for more than 15 years. At the project's onset, 400 pregnant women enrolled in the study; eligibility criteria included being less than 19 years of age, being unmarried, or being of low SES. On average, mothers assigned to the experimental condition received 9 visits during their pregnancy and 23 home visits between birth and the child's second birthday. During the home visits, information about prenatal and neonatal maternal health, childcare skills, and maternal life issues (e.g., education and employment) was provided to mothers.

Olds and colleagues have investigated short- and long-term outcomes resulting from the home visit intervention. Olds et al. (1997) and Olds, Henderson, Chamberlin, and Tatelbaum (1986) report that the intervention made an impact on maltreatment (including abuse and neglect), dependence on public assistance, multiple births in close succession, maternal criminal behavior, substance use, and child cognitive deficits. Perhaps most striking, however, are the long-term outcomes of this program. Olds et al. (1998) found that 15 years following intervention participation, there were significantly fewer arrests for the children of participating mothers in the experimental group. Furthermore, among particularly high-risk participants in the original study (as indicated by mothers being of low SES and being unmarried at childbirth), offspring of mothers in the experimental condition had lower incidence of smoking or alcohol consumption and lower rates of runaways, criminal convictions, and parole violations.

Interventions for Preschool-aged Children

Developmental changes that accompany the transition to the preschool years include an increasing use of language and physical mobility and more sophisticated, intense efforts at testing limits and asserting autonomy. The development of language skills enables children to more effectively express their needs and desires, and the development of mobility allows children to meet some of their own needs with less adult support. However, ongoing assistance from parents and caretakers is necessary for facilitating the socialization process in family and school environments. Many of the intervention programs that have been developed for preschool-aged children focus on building a strong, positive parent-child relationship and teaching specific behavior-management techniques to promote healthy child adjustment and to prevent later problems.

Webster-Stratton (1984) developed one of the most successful preventive interventions for preschool-aged children. This program involves the use of videotapes depicting a number of the most salient parenting skills for successful socialization of preschool-aged children. The program begins by focusing on the development of a positive parent-child relationship and the use of praise and rewards to encourage positive behavior. The focus then broadens to incorporate limit setting and other discipline techniques (such as time-out) and approaches to problem solving. The approach has been documented to be effective when administered in varying formats, including group and individual administration (Webster-Stratton, Hollinsworth, & Kolpacoff, 1989). Research results indicated that the program improved the parent-child interaction immediately after the intervention and one year post-intervention. Webster-Stratton has subsequently broadened the focus of the program from exclusively addressing basic parenting skills to more advanced topics, such as anger-management, communication, and self-control. These additional components have produced similarly positive effects in improving parent-child interaction and reducing child problem behavior post-treatment (Webster-Stratton, 1994). Webster-Stratton's approach has been found to be effective in samples of clinically referred children and community-based families enrolled in Head Start (Webster-Stratton, 1998).

A number of other programs have been developed specifically for families with preschool-aged children enrolled in Head Start programs. Strayhorn and Weidman (1991) developed an intervention for Head Start parents called *Parent-Child Interaction Training*, which involved teaching parents effective play skills and positive interaction and was found to produce lower teacher-ratings of problem behavior 1 year post-intervention. Peters, Bollin, and Murphy (1991) evaluated the effectiveness of a home-based program for preschool-aged children enrolled in Head Start. Home visits that addressed four domains of family functioning were conducted: education, health/nutrition/mental health, social services, and parent involvement. Research indicated that children in families who received these home visits showed improvements in the parent-child relationship and in early academic achievement when compared to children in families who did not receive home visits.

Interventions for School-aged Children

As children move into the primary school years, their social environment broadens to incorporate contexts outside of the immediate family. Consequently, interventions aimed at school-aged children typically have focused not only on supporting families and parents through an emphasis on parent training but also on addressing issues related to functioning in the school environment and in the community. Additional components of such programs include academic achievement, learning and early literacy, and parent school involvement. This is necessary because research suggests that up to 50% of children with behavior problems also have academic or learning difficulties in school (McGee et al., 1992; Moffitt, 1990).

There are several programs targeted at school-aged children with evidence of effectiveness at reducing or preventing antisocial behavior. These include the *Fast Track Program* (Conduct Problems Prevention Research Group [CPPRG], 2002a, 2002b) and the *Linking the Interests of Families and Teachers Intervention Program* (LIFT; Reid, Eddy, Fetrow, & Stoolmiller, 1999). The Fast Track Program targeted elementary school-aged children at risk for developing conduct disorders and delinquent behavior in adolescence. These children and families received a multifaceted intervention that cut across domains such as peers, the school environment, academic achievement, and the family. The family intervention component incorporated approaches to parent training shown in previous research to be effective with issues particularly relevant to the developmental needs of school-aged children. Additional emphasis was placed on parent-school involvement and early reading (CPPRG, 1992; McMahon, Slough, & CPPRG, 1996). The intervention involved weekly parent group meetings during the first-grade year and bi-weekly meetings during the second-grade year. In addition, parent-child learning activities were provided to emphasize positive parent-child interactions in a controlled environment and early literacy. Home visits and individualized programming were also utilized to address specific needs of individual families, including stress-management, marital problems, and parental depression. The results of the program evaluation indicated that at the end of first grade it successfully improved children's functioning in areas such as peer relations, emotional understanding, and reading skills. In addition, improvements in parenting were also found. In particular, parents showed less physical discipline, more consistent and appropriate discipline, and more warmth and positive involvement in their child's school (CPPRG, 1999).

The LIFT Program (Reid et al., 1999) was also designed as a preventive intervention for school-aged children at risk for antisocial behavior. LIFT utilized a cohort-sequential evaluation design in which families living in at-risk neighborhoods (in terms of low socioeconomic status) with children in the first or the fifth grade were targeted. The intervention focused on social skills and problem-solving within the school setting, behavioral parent training via parent group meetings, a behavioral program for improving playground behavior, and a telephone hotline that increased the accessibility of teachers for parents. This program has been found to be effective at decreasing aggression on the playground, increasing positive behavior one year post-intervention. Research investigating the long-term impact of the LIFT intervention is currently underway.

In addition to these programs, which involve collaboration between schools and parents, a number of preventive interventions for school-aged children have focused more exclusively on the school environment. Some of these programs have targeted children within the context of the school. For example, one program focused on improving playground behavior at recess (Barrish, Saunders, & Wolf, 1969); another involved a math and reading skills program in which the majority of children in a group needed to achieve competence using a set of skills prior to the group learning additional skills. Dolan et al. (1993) and Kellam, Rebok, Ialongo, & Mayer (1994) have reported positive impacts in both of these approaches on behavior.

Another strategy of school-based interventions has been to impact the structure of the educational environment. One such program, the School Transitional Environment Project (STEP; Felner, Brand, Adan, & Mulhall, 1993), utilized an approach in which children are divided into groups; these groups attend classes together throughout the school day in a single area of the school. Teachers in charge of each of these groups were given a broader role that includes providing counseling to children and acting as a contact within the school system for parents. An evaluation of STEP (Felner et al., 1993) demonstrated decreased dropout rates for students who participated in the intervention and increases in grades and in attendance. The dropout rates were found to be stable across time.

Interventions Involving Adolescents

Given that adolescents are typically active in social contexts that extend beyond school and family, preventive interventions for this age group have often targeted not only the school and family, but also community contexts. Some of the most compelling work with adolescents to date has involved the far end of the continuum of pathology: adolescents with extreme delinquent behavior. Chamberlain and colleagues have developed an approach called Multidimensional Treatment Foster Care (MTFC; Chamberlain & Reid, 1998; Fisher & Chamberlain, 2000). MTFC was designed to be an alternative to institutional treatment for youth with severe emotional and behavioral problems. Within the MTFC intervention, youth are placed with foster parents who have received specialized training in behavior-management techniques and who receive a high level of ongoing support and supervision from professional staff following placement. When working with youth involved with the juvenile justice system, MTFC staff members collaborate with probation officers and other justice system personnel. This approach allows troubled youth with high rates of delinquent behavior to remain in the community, with their activities and behavior closely monitored. If problems of sufficient severity occur, youth can be removed from foster homes and placed in detention. Thus, it is possible to exercise control equal to that in institutional settings while creating opportunities for youth to learn to maintain their own behavior in a more ecologically valid setting.

In addition, just as the foster home has the potential to be restrictive, it can also be significantly more flexible than typical institutional settings. Therefore, as youth demonstrate higher levels of prosocial behavior, the degree of restrictiveness in the environment can be reduced incrementally. During the time that the youth are in foster care, biological families receive intensive behavioral parent training. As youth and parents make progress in treatment, visits are initiated; these visits increase in duration over time until the parents and child are prepared for reunification. An extensive after-care program ensures that families are provided with the support necessary to be successful after the youth returns home.

The MTFC program also involves an intensive collaboration with schools. Youth carry "school cards," which are completed daily by teachers in each class, and which document the child's attendance, their completion of assignments, and the acceptability of their behavior. Program personnel are on-call to go to schools to address emergent behavior problems and to plan meetings with school personnel.

An additional emphasis of the MTFC program involves helping the youth to access and succeed in positive activities within the community. Behavioral support specialists spend time with the youth in community settings in activities such as rock climbing, arts and crafts, swimming, basketball, and basic life skills (such as shopping). Youth receive high levels of feedback regarding their behaviors in these contexts.

The MTFC approach has been evaluated via randomized trial. The approach has been shown to be effective in reducing recidivism related to delinquent behavior (Chamberlain, 1990; Chamberlain & Friman, 1997). More recently, Chamberlain and Reid (1998) reported that youth in the

MTFC had a lower incidence of substance abuse and less contact with delinquent youth than in institutional settings.

Summary of Research to Date on Preventing Antisocial Behavior

As the above review indicates, it has become increasingly clear that intervention of antisocial behavior can be effective across a broad range of ages, contexts in which the behavior occurs, and severity of the behavior. Given the difficulties encountered in past efforts to treat antisocial behavior, this is an important finding with implications for public health and social policy. However, some qualifications must me made when considering the results of prior research. For instance, although many positive effects have been documented in randomized trials, many of the studies obtained results that, while significant, are not strong effects. At the individual level, this may mean that the extent of change is more limited than would be desirable (Biglan, Ary, & Wagenaar, 2000). In addition, Eddy, Curry, and Derzon (2001) have noted that the preponderance of studies evaluating the effectiveness of preventive interventions have relied largely on self-report measures. These measures are subject to respondent bias and therefore may have limited ability to tell us whether programs are truly effective across time. Of the preventive interventions described, those that have employed hard indicators of change, such as reductions in arrest rates and other forms of criminal behavior, provide some of the most solid evidence of the effectiveness of preventive interventions.

A related concern with the prior interventions is that some efforts to treat and prevent antisocial behavior may not only be ineffective but may produce iatrogenic effects. Dishion, McCord, and Poulin (1999) describe a phenomenon regarding interventions that utilize group treatments with high-risk adolescents. These groups tended to produce higher rather than lower rates of antisocial behavior across time. The authors offer an explanation for this outcome, which they term a "deviancy training model," in which at-risk adolescents may utilize the group context to model and support antisocial behavior rather than to learn the particular skills that were the focus of the intervention.

An additional approach that was found to be problematic involved the pairing of high-risk youth with prosocial non-family members in the community in a mentor relationship. McCord (1992) reported on such a program, in which children with family problems and high-risk behavior were randomly assigned either to receive support from a social worker in their community or to receive no such support. The initial evaluation of the program showed evidence of no intervention effects. When the original participants were evaluated as they approached 50 years of age, however, those who had received the intervention had a variety of negative out-comes. McCord noted that, in these contexts, individuals who substitute for the role of family members may not be serving best those children with limited family support, if such substitution is limited in nature.

This line of research does lead to serious concerns that, until programs have been adequately evaluated and have been found to be effective, they should not be expected to produce positive change. Often, programs may seem destined to produce positive results on an intuitive basis. However, the individuals responsible for implementing these programs may take anecdotal reports of positive impact as evidence of effectiveness and may miss evidence on a larger scale suggesting ineffectiveness or iatrogenic effects. Thus, interventions must be investigated empirically. However, as we now elaborate upon, the specific manner in which interventions are developed, implemented, and then evaluated is an area that should be given further consideration; a broader range of approaches than those that have been used to date may be warranted.

From Efficacy to Effectiveness: Challenges of Dissemination

Establishing an evidence base that antisocial behavior can be prevented within the framework of randomized efficacy trials such as those described above was an important first step for the prevention field. However, be-cause most of these interventions have been evaluated under very con-trolled conditions that involved high levels of fidelity and dosage, a second stage of work has been necessary. This has involved disseminating these approaches into more typical community settings and evaluating these programs in the context of effectiveness trials. A number of promising efforts in this area are underway.

The developers of the Blueprints for Violence Prevention Program (Office of Juvenile Justice and Delinquency Prevention [OJJDP]) identified 10 preventive interventions targeted at preventing or reducing child and adolescent violence. They have developed a series of publications that de-scribe the theoretical basis for each intervention, the specific components of each intervention, the results from randomized efficacy trials provid-ing evidence of each intervention's impact, and the issues encountered in the implementation processes. A number of the interventions described earlier were included in the Blueprints program, including the prenatal home visitation intervention (Olds et al., 1986; Olds et al., 1997) and MTFC (Chamberlain, 1994; Chamberlain & Reid, 1998). In collaboration with the Center for the Study and Prevention of Violence (CSPV) at the University of Colorado, OJJDP funded an initiative to provide training and technical assistance to 50 sites around the United States to implement Blueprint programs. CSPV provided oversight and fidelity checks during the implementation process. Intervention sites were required to demonstrate adequate resources to proceed. Data are currently being gathered on the effectiveness of these implementation efforts.

Other programs with documented effectiveness have been disseminated through procedures involving training and technical assistance. In particular, the intervention for preschool-age children—developed by Webster-Stratton and colleagues (Webster-Stratton, 1994, 1998; Webster-Stratton et al., 1989)—has been implemented in multiple sites in the United States, Canada, and Europe. Providers in these communities are trained to become program trainers and, once certified, provide training and technical assistance to other community providers interested in utilizing the approach.

Despite these efforts, the ultimate success of disseminating models developed via efficacy trials remains uncertain. A number of concerns are likely to be encountered in the process. Primary among these is an issue of fidelity maintenance. As interventions developed outside of community settings are integrated into existing service delivery systems, it is uncertain whether these interventions will continue to emphasize the specific core elements shown in efficacy trials to lead to the expected outcomes. For example, an intervention involving behavioral parent training in which parents are taught effective discipline skills may not be adequately explained to providers in community service delivery programs; therefore, the program may change to conform to the community providers' preconceived approaches to intervention. Consequently, the manner in which those providers teach limit-setting skills to clientele may differ from that in the original intervention, which may impact the effectiveness of the overall intervention.

Related to fidelity is the question of whether recipients of interventions will be as easy to engage in community-based settings. Most efficacy trials provide financial compensation and other incentives to families for participating in the study. These incentives may account for high participation rates as much as any other dimension of the intervention. When such contingencies are removed, families may be less interested in participating, may skip appointments or group meetings, or may terminate treatment prematurely. All of these factors would be expected to reduce the effectiveness of an intervention.

Beyond fidelity maintenance, there is a question of the extent to which programs developed within efficacy trials will prove sustainable as community-based programs. Many of the interventions that have been shown to impact meaningful outcome variables do so at great expense.

Although economic analyses may show that the benefits of the intervention outweigh the up-front costs, it is important to recognize that these benefits accrue over the long-term, as the program recipients stay in school, are not referred for special education services, do not get arrested, and wait to have children. Thus, while from a social policy standpoint, cost effectiveness data may be important, they have little relevance to the already stressed budgets of most community and government social service agencies expected to bear the costs of the programs. Without stable funding, sustainability is highly questionable.

Beyond the financial aspects of sustainability, questions arise how programs that have relied upon high levels of expertise and staff commitment can be maintained in community settings. Many community agencies suffer from staffing shortages, high turn over and stress levels for direct service staff members, and supervisory staff members with multiple responsibilities outside of specific program activities. Limited resources make it challenging to hire and retain individuals with relevant training and experience for key positions. Thus, many of the qualities necessary to maintain a resource-intensive intervention program over time may be absent in community settings.

A final concern regarding the potential impact on communities of implementing empirically based prevention programs involves issues of ownership and empowerment. If service providers and/or families feel that interventions are being imposed upon them by outsiders and are not consistent with values in the community, there may be negative consequences. In particular, individuals may resist program elements, which may be evidenced by a lack of compliance regarding implementation on the part of providers or by a lack of acceptance of intervention components by service recipients. A related concern of bringing pre-packaged interventions into communities is that community members may perceive the prior absence of such programs as a deficit in knowledge and skills within the community. The potential to internalize or to react against deficit models is considerable, especially in communities suffering from economic disadvantage and adversity. Thus, the long-term negative impacts of dissemination in certain communities may outweigh the potential benefits.

In conclusion, although efficacy trials have been important to the field in providing an evidence base that antisocial behavior can be prevented, the value efficacy-to-effectiveness approach as the sole avenue for bringing preventive interventions to communities is less clear. Additional strategies must be developed in which community members set agendas and make critical decisions about the development and evaluation of the intervention. Within such a model, the role of the researcher shifts away from strict control over all of the elements of the intervention and evaluation to providing information that facilitates the decision-making process within communities. Perhaps most important, the primary emphasis shifts from protecting scientific principles to ensuring that the integrity of the community and its individual members are respected. Research of this nature is more emergent and organic. It is probably best to think about such research from an iterative perspective, in which specificity of the intervention and relevant outcomes come into clearer focus over time. As this process unfolds, community members may become more invested not only in the intervention, but also in the empirical evaluation of its effectiveness. Over time, the community itself may take ownership over the resolution of issues regarding tension between scientific rigor and community values.

The next section articulates how, within community-based settings, programs of this nature may be developed. In such programs, the transfer of technology regarding empirical methodology goes hand-in-hand with the development and evaluation of the intervention. Examples of several promising programs that embrace this approach are presented, and the implications of this approach taking hold in terms of the intervention content, scientific control issues, human subject issues, methodological issues, sustainability issues, and challenges to federal funding agencies are considered. Lastly, a decision-making model for future research on antisocial behavior is proposed. Within this model, the initial focus of researchers' efforts is to determine whether scientific questions requiring the efficacy-to-effectiveness approach should be the primary focus or whether community empowerment and the transfer of technology to the communities should be the primary focus. Regardless of the focus, researchers should develop alternative approaches to implementation and evaluation that protect the integrity of those communities. Such a decision-making model may facilitate the selection of appropriate designs for implementing and evaluating preventive interventions in future research on the prevention of antisocial behavior.

From "Outside-In" to "Inside-Out:" Community Empowerment Prevention Research Designs

One of the first to criticize the extent to which the prevention field had become highly reliant on randomized trials to evaluate the effectiveness of interventions was Biglan (1995), who argued that such designs insufficiently identify consistent and meaningful effects across cases. He specified a number of problems with group designs over and above those expressed in the previous section. According to Biglan, unless all cases are affected in the same manner by independent variables, group differences can be difficult to detect. Furthermore, it is possible to achieve statistical significance across multiple cases that have little value for a single case, especially when designs involve large numbers of subjects. In addition, when the unit of randomization for prevention involves larger social units (e.g., schools, neighborhoods, and communities), there are numerous additional problems of cost, quality of implementation, and lack of similarity among cases. Biglan posed the following rhetorical questions:

> Are we really willing to assume that social units like communities are alike on dimensions relevant to changing targeted cultural practices? Must we assume this? At least at this stage of our knowledge, it would seem better to approach these social units with an openness to the possibility that any given community, organization, or population is unlike any other. We can search for, identify, and verify the effects of specific independent variables on the cultural practices of those entities without having to assume that the same processes are operative in other communities or organizations. A research strategy emphasizing the need to search for and demonstrate generality is forced to include multiple cases from the outset, but such a stance detracts from exploring all contextual factors that may affect a given behavior or practice. Generalizability is not the first goal, but a goal to pursue after prediction and influence have been achieved. (p. 408)

Biglan's alternative to group designs is based on a philosophical framework called functional contextualism, which involves examining the meaning of actions in the broader milieu in which they arise. It is specifically because of the importance of context, according to Biglan, that a science oriented toward social change must shift away from individuals and toward the broader social units in which they exist (Biglan, Glasgow, & Singer, 1990). Intervention should be targeted at changing cultural practices rather than individual behavior, and methodology must similarly evaluate changes within this broader social context.

In relation to community-based interventions, Kumpfer and Hopkins (1993) noted, "the prevention field has discovered that effective preventive approaches are tailored to each at-risk group and often designed by those involved. Recent prevention approaches are designed only after thorough needs assessments are conducted, which include analysis of the family, school, peer, and community environment" (p. 15). In recent years, a number of innovative programs that utilized an approach in which work proceeded from inside the community (i.e., an inside-out model) as opposed to having been imposed by researchers from outside of the community (i.e., outside-in model) have been developed. Work by Hawkins and colleagues has been especially influential in this area, including programs such as Communities That Care (Development Research and Programs,

1994; Hawkins, Catalano, & Miller, 1992) and Preparing for the Drug-Free Years (Hawkins et al., 1988). These programs actively engaged the participating community in the design of the intervention by involving community leaders and other key stakeholders in the identification of risk and protective factors and in the selection of intervention components to be implemented.

The inside-out, community empowerment approach is especially important when designing and evaluating prevention programs involving ethnic minority groups. Despite good intentions, early prevention work in minority communities often embraced a problem-focused model of functioning, within which interventions aimed to introduce practices of the dominant culture into a community viewed as lacking (Sprott, 1994). As an alternative, recent prevention programs have been developed specifically for use with particular ethnic minority groups, including African American communities (Aktan, 1995; Aktan, Bridges, & Kumpfer, 1994a, 1994b, 1994c; Aktan, Kumpfer, & Turner, 1996; Maypole & Anderson, 1987) and Hispanic communities (Coatsworth, Szapocznik, Kurtines, & Santisteban, 1997; Szapocznik et al., 1988). Within these programs, there was an acknowledgement that unique risk factors could coexist with areas of strength particular to a specific cultural and ethnic group. Moreover, specific culturally appropriate approaches to engaging families in the intervention were used.

A project developed at the Oregon Social Learning Center, in collaboration with a Native American Tribal Head Start program (Fisher, 1998), further illustrates this approach. The Indian Family Wellness Project (IFW) has as its primary goal the development, implementation, and evaluation of a culturally specific parenting program to improve outcomes for families enrolled in the Tribal Head Start program. However, in many ways equally important to the first goal is the development of a research infrastructure within the collaborating tribal community, both to facilitate ongoing work on the IFW project and to foster the tribe's ability to develop its own research agenda. Throughout the project, now in its third year of funding, the tribe has maintained control over the decision-making process. Project staff members have worked closely with the Tribal Council, receiving tribal resolutions at critical stages in the grant development process and in the implementation of the research and intervention project components. In addition, oversight has been provided by two Tribal Council-appointed committees—one related to administrative issues and the other to cultural issues. The project has emphasized the development of a research and intervention staff consisting largely of community members, first by offering a year-long university-level research methods course to train tribal members in research methods, and more recently by providing employment and professional development opportunities to members of the tribal community. This has allowed interested community members with limited prior relevant experience and who may not have been actively involved in higher education to contribute centrally to the project.

The IFW project has also developed a tribally specific parenting curriculum using tribal stories and legends to reclaim traditional parenting methods. Finally, the project employs a multiple baseline design strategy in which the intervention was implemented at a single site, while other sites were held in baseline data collection; additional sites are being added only after there is an opportunity to evaluate the effectiveness of the intervention in a particular site.

A Decision-making Model for the Selection of Prevention Research Designs

There is no question that efficacy trials are necessary in certain circumstances. For instance, if little is known about the ability to effectively prevent the development or growth of antisocial behavior (in a particular population or in a particular context), tightly controlled studies with higher dosage levels and a greater allocation of resources may well be warranted. However, there are a variety of circumstances in which issues of scientific interest are run parallel with issues of community integrity. For instance, identifying high rates of violence in particular socioeconomically disadvantaged communities may be of great importance to the communities in question. These communities may be best served by the approach illustrated above, in which the researcher's role is more of a facilitator, helping to develop operational definitions variables, provide community members with the appropriate training and consultation to design appropriate intervention techniques and methods of evaluation, and provide input into the implementation and evaluation of the preventive intervention. The goal of this research may be less defined by strictly scientific goals and may be better conceptualized in terms of the community taking control over the systematic evaluation efforts to understand and reduce an existing problem. In this context, scientific rigor may increase over time. Moreover, if community principles are placed on par with scientific principles, community members may remain invested in the process on a long-term basis. Thus, the sustainability of scientific efforts in the community may be greatly facilitated through this approach.

With these issues in mind, a model in which the range of designs is considered at the outset of the preventive intervention project is proposed, with the suggestion that particular consideration be given to three general content areas. The first involves the locus of interest and motivation to investigate the issues in question. Projects with more scientific issues as the primary focus may be better fit for the efficacy-to-effectiveness approach. However, projects that have community-based issues as their primary focus may be better fit for the sorts of alternative approaches described above. Within this framework, relevant questions include the following:

- Was interest in the topic initiated from within the community or from outside of the community?
- If interest came from outside the community, is the investigation likely to have a negative impact on community members because of deficit models and other disempowering principles?
- If the question arises from within the community, are community members actively seeking to maintain control over the process and create products that are sustainable within the community in the long term?

A second area of consideration involves how much emphasis will be placed on disseminating the intervention (if effective) into community settings. Interventions designed for community-based settings (e.g., agencies or schools) may be best suited to be developed within those communities. This is especially true when interventions are targeted at particular groups (e.g. inner-city Latino families or lesbian and gay parents).

A third area of consideration involves how appropriate the context of the intervention to be implemented is for randomization at the individual or group level. In many contexts, especially in small communities and in communities in which individuals know each other very well, randomization at the level of the individual, and even at the group level (e.g., school or service delivery site), has the potential to create negative feelings and conflict. Perceptions that some people are receiving "special treatment" while others are being neglected often arise. In these contexts, more community-based efforts and the employment such as the multiple baseline design may be more appropriate.

Concluding Comments

This paper provides information regarding the effectiveness of programs to prevent antisocial behavior. It also provides evidence that programs clearly targeting the precursors of antisocial behavior, especially in the context of family and school/community, can prevent or slow the escalation of the development of antisocial behavior at various points along the developmental trajectory (prenatal period through adolescence). The strength of this evidence must be qualified by the fact that many of the reviewed studies report modest effect sizes and tend to rely on self-report measures. In addition, many of these studies were efficacy trials. Whether programs developed in more strictly controlled settings can be effectively disseminated in communities is still uncertain.

Perhaps more important, the field appears to be broadening in focus to acknowledge that alternatives to randomized trial designs may oftentimes be appropriate. This paper provides a conceptual framework for considering what the most effective designs are, given the circumstances and the questions under consideration. Although it is clear that efficacy-to-effectiveness is one path for the development of efforts to prevent antisocial behavior on a large scale, efforts that originate and develop from within communities will also be required to truly impact and reduce the incidence of antisocial behavior in society.

References

Ainsworth, M.D.S., Bell, S.M.V., & Stayton, D.J. (1971). Individual differences in strange-situation behavior in one-year-olds. In H.R. Schaffer (Ed.), *The origins of human social relations* (pp. 17–57). London: Academic Press.

Ainsworth, M.D.S., Bell, S.M.V., & Stayton, D.J. (1972). Individual differences in the development of some attachment behaviors. *Merrill-Palmer Quarterly, 18,* 123–43.

Aktan, G.B. (1995). Organizational frameworks of a substance use prevention program. *International Journal of Addictions, 30,* 185–201.

Aktan, G.B., Bridges, S.D., & Kumpfer, K.L. (1994a). *The Safe Haven Program: Strengthening African-American families: Children's training manual.* Detroit, MI: Detroit Department of Health, Bureau of Substance Abuse.

Aktan, G.B., Bridges, S.D., & Kumpfer, K.L. (1994b). *The Safe Haven Program: Strengthening African-American families: Family training manual.* Detroit, MI: Detroit Department of Health, Bureau of Substance Abuse.

Aktan, G.B., Bridges, S.D., & Kumpfer, K L. (1994c). *The Safe Haven Program: Strengthening African-American families: Parent training manual.* Detroit, MI: Detroit Department of Health, Bureau of Substance Abuse.

Aktan, G.B., Kumpfer, K.L., & Turner, C.W. (1996). Effectiveness of a family skills training program for substance use prevention with inner city African-American families. *Substance Use and Abuse, 31,* 157–75.

Barrish, H.H., Saunders, M., & Wolf, M.M. (1969). Good behavior game: Effects of individual contingencies for group consequences on disruptive behavior in a classroom. *Journal of Applied Behavior Analysis, 2,* 119–24.

Biglan, A. (1995). *Changing cultural practices: A contextualist framework for intervention research.* Reno, NV: Context Press.

Biglan, A., Ary, D., & Wagenaar, A.C. (2000). The value of interrupted time-series experiments for community intervention research. *Prevention Science, 1,* 34–49.

Borduin, C.M., Mann, B.J., Cone, L.T., Hengeller, S.W., Fucci, B.R., Blaske, D.M., et al. (1995). Multisystemic treatment of serious juvenile offenders: Long-term prevention of criminality and violence. *Journal of Consulting and Clinical Psychology, 63,* 569–78.

Cadoret, R.J., Yates, W.R., Throughton, E., Woodworth, G., & Stewart, M.A. (1995). Genetic-environmental interaction in the genesis of aggressivity and conduct disorders. *Archives of General Psychiatry, 52,* 916–24.

Chamberlain, P. (1990). Comparative evaluation of specialized foster care for seriously delinquent youths: A first step. *Community Alternatives: International Journal of Family Care, 2,* 21–36.

Chamberlain, P. (1994). *Family connections: Treatment foster care for adolescents with delinquency.* Eugene, OR: Castalia.

Chamberlain, P., & Friman, P.C. (1997). Residential programs for antisocial children and adolescents. In D.M. Stoff, J. Breiling, & J.D. Maser (Eds.), *Handbook of antisocial behavior* (pp. 416–24). New York: John Wiley & Sons.

Chamberlain, P., & Reid, J.B. (1998). Comparison of two community alternatives to incarceration for chronic juvenile offenders. *Journal of Consulting and Clinical Psychology, 6,* 624–33.

Coatsworth, J.D., Szapocznik, J., Kurtines, W., & Santisteban, D.E. (1997). Culturally competent psychosocial interventions with antisocial problem behavior in Hispanic youth. In D.M. Stoff, J. Breiling, & J.D. Maser (Eds.), *Handbook of antisocial behavior* (pp. 395–404). New York: John Wiley & Sons.

Cohen, P. (1993). An epidemiological study of disorders in late childhood and adolescence: I. Age- and gender-specific prevalence. *Journal of Child Psychology and Psychiatry and Allied Disciplines, 34,* 851–67.

Conduct Problems Prevention Research Group. (1992). A developmental and clinical model for the prevention of conduct disorders: The FAST Track program. *Development and Psychopathology, 4,* 509–27.

Conduct Problems Prevention Research Group. (2002a). The implementation of the Fast Track Program: An example of a large-scale prevention science efficacy trial. *Journal of Abnormal Child Psychology, 30*(1), 1–17.

Conduct Problems Prevention Research Group. (2002b). Evaluation of the first 3 years of the Fast Track prevention trial with children at high risk for adolescent conduct problems. *Journal of Abnormal Child Psychology, 30*(1), 19–35.

Development Research & Programs. (1994). *Communities That Care planning kit.* Seattle: Author.

DiLalla, L.F., & Gottesman, I.I. (1989). Heterogeneity of cause for delinquency and criminality: Lifespan perspectives. *Development and Psychopathology, 1,* 339–49.

Dishion, T.J., French, D.C., & Patterson, G.R. (1995). The development and ecology of antisocial behavior. In D. Cicchetti & D.J. Cohen (Eds.), *Developmental psychopathology. Vol 2: Risk, disorder & adaptation* (pp. 421–71). NYC: Wiley & Sons.

Dishion, T.J., McCord, J., & Poulin, F. (1999). When interventions harm: Peer groups and problem behavior. *American Psychologist, 54,* 755–64.

Dodge, K.A., Pettit, G.S., Bates, J.E., & Valente, E. (1995). Social information-processing patterns partially mediate the effect of early physical abuse on later conduct problems. *Journal of Abnormal Psychology, 104,* 632–43.

Dodge, K.A., & Schwartz, D. (1997). Social information processing mechanisms in aggressive behavior. In D.M. Stoff, & J. Breiling (Eds.), *Handbook of antisocial behavior* (pp. 171–80). NYC: Wiley & Sons.

Dolan, L.J., Kellam, S.G., Brown, C.H., Werthamer-Larsson, L., Rebok, G.W., Mayer, L.S., et al. (1993). The short-term impact of two classroom-based preventive interventions on aggressive and shy behaviors and poor achievement. *Journal of Applied Developmental Psychology, 14*, 317–45.

Eddy, J.M., Curry, V., & Derzon, J. (2001). *Youth antisocial behavior and substance abuse: Interrelationship and empirically-based interventions.* Manuscript submitted for publication.

Farrington, D.P. (1995). The 12th Jack Tizard memorial lecture. The development of offending and antisocial behaviour from childhood: Key findings from the Cambridge Study in Delinquent Development. *Journal of Child Psychology and Psychiatry, 360*, 929–64.

Felner, R.D., Brand, S., Adan, A.M., Mulhall, P.F., Flowers, N., Sartain, B., & DuBois, D.L. (1993). Restructuring the ecology of the school as an approach to prevention during school transitions: Longitudinal follow-ups and extensions of the school transitional environment project (STEP). *Prevention in Human Services 10* (2), 103–36.

Fingerhut, L.A., & Kleinman, J.C. (1990). International and interstate comparisons of homicides among young males. *Journal of the American Medical Association, 263*, 3292–95.

Fisher, P.A. (1998). *Indian Wellness Preventive Intervention Project* (Grant number 1 R01 DA 12231). Washington, DC: National Institute on Drug Abuse, Prevention Research Branch, Division of Epidemiology and Prevention Research.

Fisher, P.A., & Chamberlain, P. (2000). Multidimensional treatment foster care: A program for intensive parenting, family support, and skill building. *Journal of Emotional and Behavioral Disorders, 8*, 155–64.

Gottesman, I.I., & Goldsmith, H.H. (1994). Developmental psychopathology of antisocial behavior: Inserting genes into its ontogenesis and epigenesis. In C.A. Nelson (Ed.), *Threats to optimal development: Integrating biological, psychological, & social risk factors. The Minnesota symposium on child psychology* (Vol. 27, pp. 69–104). Hillsdale, NJ: Lawrence Erlbaum.

Greenberg, M.T., Kusche, C.A., Speltz, M. (1991). Emotional regulation, self-control, and psychopathology: The role of relationships in early childhood. In D. Cicchetti & S. Toth (Eds.), *Internalizing and externalizing expressions of dysfunction* (pp. 21–55). Hillsdale, NJ: Lawrence Erlbaum.

Greenwood, P.W., Model, K.E., Rydell, C.P., & Chiesa, J. (1996). *Diverting children from a life of crime: Measuring costs and benefits.* Santa Monica, CA: Rand.

Hawkins, J.D., Catalano, R.F., Brown, E.O., Vadasy, P.F., Roberts, C., Fitzmahan, D., et al. (1988). *Preparing for the drug (free) years: A family activity book.* Seattle: Comprehensive Health Education Foundation.

Hawkins, J.D., Catalano, R.F., & Miller, J.Y. (1992). Risk and protective factors for alcohol and other drug problems in adolescence and early adulthood: Implications for substance abuse prevention. *Psychological Bulletin, 112*, 64–105.

Hirschi, T. (1969). *Causes of delinquency.* Berkeley: University of California.

Hogue, A., & Liddle, H.A. (1999). Family-based preventive intervention: An approach to preventing substance use and antisocial behavior. *American Journal of Orthopsychiatry, 69*, 278–93.

Kellam, S.G., Rebok, G.W., Ialongo, N., & Mayer, L.S. (1994). The course and malleability of aggressive behavior from early first grade into middle school: Results of a developmental epidemiologically-based preventive trial. *Journal of Child Psychology and Psychiatry, 35*, 259–81.

Kochanska, G. (1997). Mutually responsive orientation between mothers and their young children: Implications for early socialization. *Child Development, 68*, 94–112.

Kochanska, G. (1998). Mother-child relationship, child fearfulness, and emerging attachment: A short-term longitudinal study. *Developmental Psychology, 34*, 480–90.

Kumpfer, K.L., & Hopkins, R. (1993). Prevention: Current research and trends. *Recent Advances in Addictive Disorders, 16*, 11–20.

Loeber, R. (1982). The stability of antisocial and delinquent child behavior: A review. *Psychological Bulletin, 53,* 1431–46.

Maypole, D.E., & Anderson, R.B. (1987). Culture-specific substance abuse prevention for Blacks. *Community Mental Health Journal, 23,* 135–39.

McCord, J. (1992). The Cambridge-Somerville Study: A pioneering longitudinal-experimental study of delinquency prevention. In J. McCord & R.E. Tremblay (Eds.), *Preventing antisocial behavior: Interventions from birth through adolescence* (pp. 196–206). New York: Guilford Press.

McGee, R., Feehan, M., Williams, S., & Anderson, J. (1992). DSM-III disorders from age 11 to age 15 years. *Journal of the American Academy of Child and Adolescent Psychiatry, 31,* 50–59.

McMahon, R.J., Slough, N., & the Conduct Problems Prevention Research Group (1996). Family-based intervention in the FAST Track Program. In R.D. Peters & R.J. McMahon (Eds.), *Preventing childhood disorders, substance abuse, and delinquency* (pp. 90–110). Thousand Oaks, CA: Sage.

Moffitt, T.E. (1990). Juvenile delinquency and attention deficit disorder: Boys' developmental trajectories from age 3 to age 15. *Child Development, 61,* 893–910.

Moffitt, T.E. (1993). Adolescence-limited and life-course-persistent antisocial behavior: A developmental taxonomy. *Psychological Review, 100,* 674–701.

Neiderhiser, J.M., Reiss, D., & Hetherington, E.M. (1996). Genetically informative designs for distinguishing developmental pathways during adolescence: Responsible and antisocial behavior. *Development and Psychopathology, 8,* 779–91.

Offord, D.R., Boyle, M.C., & Racine, Y.A. (1991). The epidemiology of antisocial behavior in childhood and adolescence. In D.J. Peplar & K.H. Rubin (Eds.), *The development and treatment of childhood aggression* (pp. 31–54). Hillsdale, NJ: Lawrence Erlbaum.

Olds, D., Eckenrode, J., Henderson, C.R., Kitzman, H., Powers, J., Cole, R., et al. (1997). Long-term effects of home visitation on maternal life-course and child abuse and neglect: Fifteen-year follow-up of a randomized trial. *Journal of the American Medical Association, 278,* 637–43.

Olds, D., Henderson, C., Chamberlin, R., & Tatelbaum, R. (1986). Preventing child abuse and neglect: A randomized trial of nurse home visitation. *Pediatrics, 78,* 65–78.

Olds, D., Henderson, C., Cole, R., Eckenrode, J., Kitzman, H., Luckey, D., et al. (1998). Long-term effects of nurse home visitation on children's criminal and antisocial behavior: 15-year follow-up of a randomized controlled trial. *Journal of the American Medical Association, 280,* 1238–44.

Olds, D., Henderson, C.R., Tatelbaum, R., & Chamberlin, R. (1988). Improving the life-course development of socially disadvantaged mothers: A randomized trial of nurse home visitation. *American Journal of Public Health, 78,* 1436–45.

Olds, D., & Korfmacher, J. (1997). Home visitation [Special issue]. *Journal of Community Psychology, 1,* 25.

Olweus, D. (1979). Stability of aggressive reaction patterns in males: A review. *Psychological Bulletin, 86,* 852–75.

Patterson, G.R. (1982). *Coercive family process.* Eugene, OR: Castalia.

Patterson, G.R., Capaldi, D.M., & Bank, L. (1991). An early starter model predicting delinquency. In D.J. Pepler & K.H. Rubin (Eds.), *The development and treatment of childhood aggression* (pp. 139–68). Hillsdale, NJ: Lawrence Erlbaum.

Patterson, G.R., DeBaryshe, B.D., & Ramsey, E. (1989). A developmental perspective on antisocial behavior [Special issue]. *American Psychologist, 44,* 329–35.

Patterson, G.R., & Fisher, P.A. (2002). Recent developments in our understanding of parenting: Bidirectional effects, causal models, and the search for parsimony. In M. Bornstein (Ed.),

Handbook of parenting: Practical and applied parenting (2nd ed., Vol. 5, pp. 59–88). Mahwah, NJ: Erlbaum.

Patterson, G.R., Reid, J.B., & Dishion, T.J. (1992). *Antisocial boys: A social learning approach. Vol. 4.* Eugene, OR: Castalia.

Peters, D.L., Bollin, G.G., & Murphy, R.E. (1991). Head Start's influence on parental competence and child competence. In S.B. Silvern (Ed.), *Advances in reading/language research: A research annual, Vol. 5: Literacy through family, community, and school interaction* (pp. 91–123). Greenwich, CT: Jai Press.

Plomin, R., Nitz, K., & Rowe, D.C. (1990). Behavioral genetics and aggressive behavior in childhood. In M. Lewis & S.M. Miller (Eds.), *Handbook of developmental psychopathology* (pp. 119–33). New York: Plenum Press.

Reid, J.B. (1993). Prevention of conduct disorder before and after school entry: Relating interventions to development findings. *Journal of Development and Psychopathology, 5,* 243–62.

Reid, J.B., & Eddy, J.M. (1997). The prevention of antisocial behavior: Some considerations in the search for effective interventions. In D.M. Stoff, J. Breiling, & J.D. Maser (Eds.), *Handbook of antisocial behavior* (pp. 343–356) NYC: Wiley & Sons.

Reid, J.B., Eddy, J.M., Fetrow, R.A., & Stoolmiller, M. (1999). Description and immediate impacts of a preventative intervention for conduct problems. *American Journal of Community Psychology, 24,* 483–517.

Reid, J.B., & Patterson, G.R. (1989). The development of antisocial behavior patterns in childhood and adolescence. *European Journal of Personality, 3,* 107–19.

Robins, L.N. (1981). Epidemiological approaches to natural history research: Antisocial disorders in children. *Journal of the American Academy of Child Psychiatry, 20,* 566–80.

Shaw, D.S., Bell, R.Q., & Gilliom, M. (2000). A truly early starter model of antisocial behavior revisited. *Clinical Child & Family Psychology Review, 3,* 155–72.

Sickmund, M., Snyder, H.N., & Poe-Yamagata, E. (1997). *Juvenile offenders and victims: 1997 update on violence.* Pittsburgh, PA: National Center for Juvenile Justice.

Snyder, H., & Sickmund, M. (1995). *Juvenile offenders and victims: A national report.* Washington, DC: U.S. Department of Justice, Office of Justice Problems, Office of Juvenile Justice and Delinquency Prevention.

Sprott, J.E. (1994). One person's "spoiling" is another's freedom to become: Overcoming ethnocentric views about parental control. *Social Science and Medicine, 38,* 1111–24.

Smith, P.B., & Pederson, D.R. (1988). Maternal sensitivity and patterns of infant-mother attachment. *Child Development, 59,* 1097–01.

Sroufe, L.A. (1983). Infant-caregiver attachment and patterns of adaptation in pre-school: The roots of maladaptation and competence. In M. Perlmutter (Ed.), *Minnesota symposium in child psychology* (Vol. 16, pp. 41–81). Hillsdale, NJ: Lawrence Erlbaum.

Strayhorn, J.M., & Weidman, C. (1991) Follow-up one year after parent-child interaction training: effects on behavior of preschool children. *Journal of the American Academy of Child and Adolescent Psychiatry, 30,* 138-43.

Szapocznik, J., Perez-Vidal, A., Brickman, A.L., Foote, F.H., Santisteban, D., & Hervis, O. (1988). Engaging adolescent drug abusers and their families in treatment: A strategic structural systems approach. *Journal of Consulting and Clinical Psychology, 56,* 552–57.

Webster-Stratton, C. (1984). Randomized trial of two parent-training programs for families with conduct disordered children. *Journal of Consulting and Clinical Psychology, 52,* 666–78.

Webster-Stratton, C. (1994). Advancing videotape parent training: A comparison study. *Journal of Consulting and Clinical Psychology, 62,* 583–93.

Webster-Stratton, C. (1998). Preventing conduct problems in Head Start children: Strengthening parenting competencies. *Journal of Consulting and Clinical Pscyhology, 66,* 715–30.

Webster-Stratton, C., Hollinsworth, T., & Kolpacoff, M. (1989). The long-term effectiveness and clinical significance of three cost-effective training programs for families with conduct problem children. *Journal of Consulting and Clinical Psychology, 57*, 550–53.

Wolff, S. (1961). Social and family background of pre-school children with behaviour disorders attending a child guidance clinic. *Journal of Child Psychology & Psychiatry, 2*, 260–68.

World Health Organization (1992). *Annual report on homicide*. Geneva, Switzerland: Author.

Chapter 2

Causal Structure of Alcohol Use and Problems in Early Life

Multilevel Etiology and Implications for Prevention

Robert A. Zucker

This is a chapter that examines the causes of adolescent alcohol use and abuse. Alcohol is a unique drug. It's the nation's most commonly abused drug, yet it can have some healthful benefits and is a part of many common cultural rituals. At the same time, its use is associated with a number of costly problems. This chapter will discuss alcohol's unique status and explore the factors influencing the development of alcohol abuse. We will give special attention to the relationship between behavioral under-control and alcohol abuse, as well as the inter-relation of risk factors of abuse. Finally, the implications of our understanding of the development of alcohol abuse on prevention efforts are discussed.

The Special Nature of Alcohol as a Drug

The High Prevalence of Alcohol Problems

Alcohol is the nation's most common drug of abuse. Although the popular myth is that the harder drugs form the bulk of the nation's drug problems, both the Epidemiologic Catchment Area (ECA) study (Regier et al., 1990), as well as the more recent National Comorbidity Study (NCS; Kessler et al., 1994), indicate otherwise. (See Table 1.) The NCS United States population

**Table 1. Lifetime and 12-Month Prevalence of DSM-III-R
Substance Use Disorders Estimated U.S. Population Rates**

Disorder	Lifetime	12 Month
Any substance use disorder	26.6	11.3
Alcohol dependent	14.1	7.2
Alcohol abuse only	9.4	2.5
Any alcohol disorder	23.5	9.7
Other drug dependence	7.5	2.8
Other drug abuse	4.4	0.8
Any other drug disorder	11.9	3.6
Any other drug disorder without alcohol disorder	3.1	1.6

Note: Data is adapted from "Lifetime and 12-month Prevalence of DSM-III-R Psychiatric Disorders in the United States," by R.C. Kessler et al., 1994, *Archives of General
Psychiatry, 51*, 8–19 and are DSM-III-R diagnoses for persons aged 15–54 years in the
non-institutionalized population.

estimates show that one in four individuals (26.6%) have had a substance
use disorder at some point in their lives. The rate of those with an active
diagnosis over the past year is one in nine. The lifetime prevalence rate for
those with an "other drug" diagnosis but no alcohol diagnosis is only 1 in
32 (3.1%), and the 12-month rate is only 1 in 62. To recast these data, among
those who have had any substance use disorder, 88% have had an alcohol
diagnosis, either with or without an "other drug" diagnosis. This pattern
is evident even at the more severe diagnostic level of dependence; here
82% of those with a dependence diagnosis are either alcohol dependent
or alcohol and other drug dependent (Kessler et al., 1994; Kessler, Crum,
Warner, Nelson, Schulenberg, & Anthony, 1997).

   Although these data describe rates of individual disorder in the adult
subpopulation, when they are recast according to a life course perspective, they describe one of the end points that prevention programming
ultimately needs to address: the extraordinarily high level of this set of
problems in the adult population. Given what is known about the emergence and widespread nature of these problems in adolescence and pread-
olescence, the adult data are also an indirect indicator of their apparent
persistence. Evaluating these data from still another perspective, among
that subset of the adult population where alcohol use disorders (AUD) are
present, it is reasonable to anticipate that parenting will, to some degree,
be impaired.

   Other data make this case more directly, and again indicated that the
child risk for family exposure to drugs of abuse is most heavily exposure to alcohol use disorders. Data from the 1996 Substance Abuse and
Mental Health Services Administration (SAMHSA) National Household

Survey on Drug Abuse (Huang, Cerbone, & Gfroerer, 1998) provide an estimate of the magnitude of the problem as it impinges upon children. The report also addresses the issue of "what drug." Projections from the SAMHSA national sample are that 6.2 million children, or approximately 8.3% of children in the United States, are living in households where one or more of the parents have been actively alcohol dependent in the past year. (See Table 2.) When the risk structure is defined as parents who are dependent upon illicit drugs as well as alcohol, the figure increases to 10.0%. (See Table 3.) In other words, 83% of significantly drug-involved families are dealing with alcohol dependence either as the only drug of choice, or one of the primary drugs of choice. Other drug involvement implicates only 17% of the population. Although these figures are familiar to epidemiologists, they are not common knowledge either in the popular press or among policymakers, where drug dependence and its impact upon children is more often characterized as a problem of illicit drug use.

Table 2. Estimated Number and Percentage of Children[1] in the Household[2] with at Least One Parent Dependent on Alcohol, by Children's Ages: NHSDA 1996 (Johnston, O'Malley, & Bachman, 1997)

Children's age in years	Estimated population 17 years or younger	Estimated population 17 years or younger who had at least one parent dependent on alcohol	Percentage of population 17 years or younger who had at least one parent dependent on alcohol
Under 2	8,590,119	678,923	7.9
2–5	18,766,120	1,551,952	8.3
6–9	18,333,494	1,616,156	8.8
10–13	15,015,264	1,225,437	8.2
14–17	13,801,727	1,115,056	8.1
Total	**74,506,723**	**6,187,524**	**8.3**

[1]Children are defined as biological, step, adoptive, or foster.

[2]Children aged 17 years and less and not living with at least one parent for most of the quarter of the NHSDA interview have been excluded from this analysis. According to the March 1995 Current Population Survey (Substance Abuse and Mental Health Services Administration, 1996), this amounts to approximately 3 million (or 4%) of children under 18 years of age.

Note: Alcohol dependence is determined by two responses: alcohol was used in the past year and the user reported meeting three of the following six DSM-IV dependence criteria: built up a tolerance for alcohol; used alcohol more often than intended; wanted or tried to cut down on alcohol use, but found they couldn't; had a month or more in the past year when spent a great deal of time getting the alcohol, using alcohol, or recovering from its effects; alcohol reduced participation in important activities; alcohol caused emotional or health problems.

Source: Adapted from Preliminary Results from the 1997 National Household Survey on Drug Abuse: Population Estimates, 1995, by Substance Abuse and Mental Health Services Administration, 1996.

Table 3. Estimated Number and Percentage of Children[1] in the Household[2]
with at Least One Parent Dependent on Alcohol and/or Illicit Drugs, by
Children's Ages: National Household Survey on Drug Abuse, 1996
(Johnston, O'Malley, & Bachman, 1997)

Children's age in years	Estimated population 17 years or younger	Estimated population 17 years or less with at least one parent dependent on alcohol and/or illicit drugs	Percent of population 17 years or less with at least one parent dependent on alcohol and/or illicit drugs
Under 2	8,590,119	867,674	10.1
2–5	18,766,120	1,884,394	10.0
6–9	18,333,494	1,912,796	10.4
10–13	15,015,264	1,464,345	9.8
14–17	13,801,727	1,353,769	9.8
Total	74,506,723	7,482,978	10.0

[1]Children are defined as biological, step, adoptive, or foster.

[2]Children aged 17 years and less and not living with at least one parent for most of the quarter of the NHSDA interview have been excluded from this analysis. According to the March 1995 Current Population Survey (Substance Abuse & Mental Health Services Administration, 1996), this amounts to approximately 3 million (or 4%) of children under 18 years of age.

Note: Substance dependence is defined as dependence on alcohol and/or one or more illicit drugs. It is determined by two responses: alcohol was used in the past year and the user reported meeting three of the following six DSM-IV dependence criteria: built up a tolerance for the substance; used the substance more often than intended; wanted or tried to cut down on substance use, but found they couldn't; had a month or more in the past year when spent a great deal of time getting the substance, using it, or recovering from its effects; the substance reduced participation in important activities; the substance caused emotional or health problems.

Source: Adapted from *Preliminary Results from the 1997 National Household Survey on Drug Abuse: Population Estimates*, 1995, by Substance Abuse and Mental Health Services Administration, 1996.

Cultural Ambivalence Toward Alcohol

Although alcohol consumption is illegal in adolescence, alcohol becomes a legal drug at age 21. Not only does it become legal, among users, alcohol also tends to be considered a "good" drug. It has been touted for its cardio-vascular protective effects; it is a drug that most of the mainstream culture enjoys, using it for celebration, leisure, courting, and mourning. Alcohol has been described as the world's most domesticated drug (Zucker, 2000). Unlike tobacco, where effects are uniformly negative, and the entire spectrum of illicit drugs, ethanol occupies a special niche. Because of the regulated nature of its use, the ability to drink legally has commonly been a marker of the achievement of adult status (Maddox & McCall, 1964), and the binge drinking that often takes place at age 21 has become a rite of passage in certain groups. More generally, adolescents see alcohol use as a socially desirable activity. They constantly value it for its positive effects in social situations (Schulenberg, Maggs, Long et al., 2001) and tend to ignore the negative consequences of its use (Maggs, 1997). In addition, in normal samples, it is not necessarily related to poorer antecedent functioning. For example, in a prospective study beginning with children in second through 4th grade, Hops, Davis, and Lewin (1999) found that positive social behavior with peers, as well as family conflict (for girls), were predictive of alcohol use (but not alcohol and other drug involvement) when the children were teenagers.

The proven protective effects of moderate alcohol consumption on the cardiovascular system (Garg, Wagener, & Madens, 1993; Klatsky, 1994; Miller, Beckles, Maude, & Carson, 1990), combined with the drug's legality and social utility (Klein, 1991), make it likely that campaigns to eliminate use will be ineffective at best, and generate community antagonism at worst, in regions of the country where drinking is more prevalent. Thus, implementation of prevention programming aimed at changing patterns of use with alcohol need to take careful account of the anomalous place that this drug occupies.

The Development of Alcohol Use and Alcohol Problems

Because the use of alcohol becomes legal at age 21, it is reasonable to expect that a developmental boundary period will exist, where increasing portions of the population will use the drug as they approach 21. Approximately 80% of high school seniors use alcohol to some degree (Johnston, O'Malley, and Bachman, 1997). Table 4 illustrates this age progression, both of use

Table 4. Grade of First Alcohol Use and Drunkenness as Retrospectively Reported by Tenth Grade Students (Percentage of U.S. Population)

	Grade in school	Approximate age	Use	Cumulative use	First use of alcohol	Cumulative population
Grade school	4	10	5.5	5.5	1.1	1.1
	5	11	3.6	9.1	1.0	2.1
	6	12	7.0	16.1	2.5	4.6
Middle school	7	13	12.3	28.4	6.4	11.0
	8	14	18.3	46.7	11.2	22.2
High school	9	15	17.1	63.8	16.6	38.8
	10	16	6.8	70.6	8.1	46.9
	11		No data collected			
	12	18		80.7		63.2

Note: The definition of a drink changed in 1993 to "more than a few sips" so that national estimates from data collected after 1993 are slightly lower than in earlier reports.

Source: Data is 1995 survey data adapted from National Survey Results on Drug Use from Monitoring The Future Study, 1975–1995: Vol. 1: Secondary School Students, by L.D. Johnston, P.M. O'Malley & J.G. Bachman, 1997.

and of the problem indicator drunkenness. As illustrated by the low-end figures, there are substantial individual differences, with 6% of the population using at age 10, even though the median age of first use is 14, and 1% having already experienced drunkenness by age 10, even though the median age for this is 17 years. Gender differences are negligible when the indicator is use, but there is typically some differentiation among problem indicators, with boys showing substantially higher problem levels than girls.

Recent national epidemiologic data on alcohol use and onset of alcohol use disorders (Grant, 1997) also indicate that social change has produced increasingly earlier ages of first use, as well as an increasing proportion of the population who receive an AUD diagnosis. Furthermore, there is substantial evidence for gender homogenization of problems during the interval from the turn of the last century to the 1990s. For persons born around the turn of the last century, males were 2.4 times more likely to use alcohol and were 4.9 times more likely to achieve an AUD diagnosis at some point in their lives. For persons born during the Vietnam era, the comparable figures are 1.2 and 1.4 (Grant, 1997).

Alcohol is a problem drug. Earlier and heavier use have been causally linked to the presence of a behavioral cluster including both delinquent activity and poorer school performance. The proximal, as well as distal, variables contributing to these effects are not fully understood. A significant finding of the past generation has been the link between the normative activities of adolescence and involvement with alcohol. Using a primarily social-psychologist theory base called Problem Behavior Therapy, Jessor and Jessor (1997) assembled an impressive empirical base, heavily replicated by other investigators, which has proposed that the normative patterns of adolescence—increasing independence from parents; valuing independence over achievement, peers over parents, and rebellion over conformity—cohere as a system. The syndrome precedes the onset of alcohol use, predicts the onset of problem use, and forecasts a cluster of problem behaviors. These behaviors include an increasing involvement with alcohol, progression into other drugs (particularly marijuana), poorer school performance, an earlier transition into sexual activity (Jessor, Costa, Jessor, & Donovan, 1983; Jessor & Jessor, 1975) and involvement in other social norm breaking (i.e., delinquent) behavior (Donovan & Jessor, 1985; Jessor & Jessor, 1977; Kandel, 1978). Investigators have documented the mediational role played by increasing involvement with peers (Dishion & Loeber, 1985; Dishion, Patterson, & Reid, 1988), but have also shown that parent socialization influences continue to play an indirect role by overseeing the choice of peers (Blanton, Gibbons, Gerrard, Conger, & Smith, 1997; Jacob & Leonard,

1994) and monitoring patterns of activity with peers (Andrews, Hops, & Duncan, 1997; Ary, Tildesley, Hops, & Andrews, 1993; Wills & Cleary, 1996).

Although the empirical work generated by problem behavior theory has focused primarily on the role of the perceived environment and the importance of expectancies as instigators of social behavior, the theory is both a social-psychological theory, as well as a social-structural theory. In fact, one of the most important parts of the theory has been the proposition that the emergence of problem behavior itself is normative to this particular developmental period, and when the normative control structure of young adulthood emphasizes different values and provides different controls, the deviance will begin to decrease. In recent work by Jessor and his colleagues (Jessor, Donovan, & Costa, 1991), the proximal importance of real differences in social structure as stimulators or dampeners of social behavior has been addressed, and some empirical support for this sociologically appealing proposition has been demonstrated. Jessor et al. (1991) examined changes in alcohol use and problems, as well as a number of other indicators of the problem behavior syndrome, over two intervals: from junior high school to young adulthood in one sample and from the freshman year of college into the last 20s for the other. Among the results were three findings: Conventionality increased during these intervals, the greatest increases were among those who were more problem-prone in adolescence, and there is a continued association of alcohol abuse with a more general composite deviance syndrome. So, on the one hand, alcohol problems continue to be empirically linked with other indicators of delinquent/antisocial behavior (Donovan & Jessor, 1985), and on the other hand, changes in role demands brought about changes in patterns of alcohol use.

It has not always been recognized that much of the prevention work of the last decade owes its origins to this theoretical base. For example, the observation that youth overestimate the actual prevalence of all forms of substance use by peers and adults (Hansen, 1988) is derivative from the Jessors' work emphasizing the importance of the perceived as compared to the actual environment in regulating social behavior (Jessor & Jessor, 1977). Similarly, the design of norm setting interventions as a method to delay onset of alcohol use (Donaldson, Graham, & Hansen, 1995; MacKinnon et al., 1991) is attributable to this body of work. The existing evidence, at least during early adolescence, has shown the effectiveness of correcting adolescents' overestimates (i.e., resetting the norms), with norm setting serving as a mediator of lower problem use (e.g., drunkenness, drinking more than planned; Wynn, Schulenberg, Maggs, & Zucker, 2000). The Wynn et al. data suggest that this procedure is not uniformly effective across grade levels, with stronger effects being shown at 8th grade (around age 14, when the majority of students have already begun to use), rather than at earlier grade levels.

Even more recently, Project Northland, the largest scale community trial designed to reduce both onset and problem use of alcohol (Wagenaar & Perry, 1995), has used problem behavior theory (Perry & Jessor, 1985), as well as social-epidemiological concepts, to design a multilevel program directed at individual, familial, and community level targets. This program, focused initially on 6th graders—a time when national norms would suggest that only 20% of youth will have begun use and where only 6% will have some problem use (see Table 4)—from 24 school districts in northeast Minnesota, has worked to manipulate both supply and demand (Williams, Perry, Farbakhsh, & Veblen-Mortenson, 1999). The supply reduction protocol involved an extensive menu of community action task forces, forums, and media programs aimed at changing community norms about alcohol; increasing availability of alternative alcohol-free activities; and raising community consciousness about access and availability. Demand reduction programming targeted the adolescents and their families; in addition to providing school programming to teach refusal skills, facilitate parent-child communication, and guide students into more alcohol-free alternative activities. Early results, based on onset data, reports of frequency of use, as well as scores on problem-proneness scales, indicate greater impact on initial non-users and on those with lower risk behavioral profiles, but with some effect also on higher risk subpopulations (Perry et al., 1996; Williams et al., 1999). At the same time, a stance of cautious optimism needs to be adopted toward this massive program and database given the complexity of its design and the necessary incompleteness of analysis at this stage of the project's work.

Another recent program stemming from this theory base is highly relevant in understanding patterns of drinking variability over time. This work, by Schulenberg and colleagues (Schulenberg, Maggs, Long et al., 2001; Schulenberg & Maggs, 2002; Schulenberg, O'Malley, Bachman, Wadsworth, & Johnston, 1996; Schulenberg, Wadsworth, O'Malley, Bachman, & Johnston, 1996), picks up on the Jessor group's proposition that patterns of alcohol use vary with developmental role structure. However, Schulenberg's group also provides evidence that there is considerable heterogeneity among population subgroups even within the same role structure.

Using national panel data from the Monitoring the Future (MTF) project, one group (Bachman, Wadsworth, O'Malley, Johnston, & Schulenberg, 1997; Johnston, O'Malley, & Bachman, 1997) demonstrated that during the period from ages 18 to 25, the rate of binge drinking (having 5 or more drinks in a row at least twice in the past two weeks) for college students in 4-year residential colleges as compared to others was higher. However, with a change to post-college life, the rates converge (Schulenberg & Maggs, 2002; Schulenberg, Maggs, Steinman, & Zucker, 2001). In other words, the social structure provided a moratorium from role demands (e.g., job, marriage) which permitted drinking to excess. Once this protective structure is not available, environmental contingencies provide many more penalties for excessive drinking and bingeing rates drop to the level found among those who did not have this time-out.

In addition to this structural main effect, two other studies using MTF data describe the substantial heterogeneity that exists in patterns of stability and change in frequent binge drinking between ages 18 and 24. Using biennial assessments of drinking and related psychosocial variation, six distinct trajectories of binge drinking were identified that accounted for over 90% of the sample and that included stable patterns (Never, Rare, and Chronic) as well as patterns of cross temporal variation (Decreased, Increased, and Fling; Schulenberg, O'Malley et al., 1996). Females were over-represented in the Never group, and underrepresented in the Chronic and Increased groups. Binge trajectory differences were related to concomitant variation in problems with alcohol, attitudes about heavy drinking, time spent with heavily drinking peers, and extent of illicit drug involvement. In other words, a pattern of behaviors was being indexed by the binge variation, but it encompassed a substantially larger set of characteristics that shifted (or remained stable) along with the drinking. Furthermore, being lower in conventionality and self-efficacy, as well as drinking to get drunk, were senior year risk factors for membership in the Increased trajectory group, while higher self-efficacy and lower intent of drinking to get drunk were protective factors against involvement in the continued bingeing trajectory among initially frequent binge drinkers (Schulenberg, Wadsworth et al., 1996).

The similarities and differences between Chronic binge drinkers and the Decreased group are also of special interest. One group sustained a pattern of heavy bingeing throughout the years between ages 18 to 24; the other's problem use dropped to a non-problem level (Schulenberg, Wadsworth et al., 1996). Both groups started with high rates of problem use at the end of high school. Both groups had high levels of antisociality/alienation, used drinking as a way of coping, had high expectations of future use, along with low GPAs and low levels of conventionality. However, protective factors against continued drinking (the Decreased Group) were being female, having higher self-efficacy, and more work role readiness, doing less "effect" drinking (drinking to get drunk), and having greater loneliness (p. 667). Schulenberg and colleagues suggest this latter

characteristic may be a marker of less satisfaction of senior year social relationships. It may also indirectly indicate dissatisfaction with membership
in the college drinking groups that form the base for social relationships.
Of special interest is that the activity profile for the Chronic group is consistent with the pattern described by the Jessor group for early onset and
problem use in adolescence. Also interesting is the parallelism between the
Chronic group and Weber and colleagues' (Weber, Graham, Hansen, Flay, &
Anderson, 1989) problem prone early onset adolescents.

We return to this point below. For the moment, the consistency of
behavioral patterning of the high problem group across several developmental transitions raises the issue of what is ultimately causal and what is
a proximal marker of a longer-term process.

Factors Influencing the Development of Alcohol Abuse: A Multilevel Causal Structure

The Role of Behavioral Undercontrol

A robust group of studies spanning the interval from very early childhood to adulthood strongly implicate behavioral undercontrol as a factor
precursive to the adult outcomes of alcohol abuse and dependence. Adult
clinical data support this set of findings: the strongest comorbid association
of alcoholism with other psychiatric disorders is the connection between
alcoholism and antisocial personality disorder. Among men, the odds ratio is 12:1; among women, it is 29:1 (Kessler et al., 1997). A parallel line
of reasoning to problem behavior theory has been that individual differences in temperament—probably mediated by genetics and pertaining to
high activity level, low attention span and behavioral undercontrol—are
an earlier link in the chain of risk for alcohol use and later childhood and
adolescence problems. The temperament substrate, when coupled with an
environmental structure that facilitates the development of these initially
neutral temperamental attributes, is hypothesized to culminate in a behavioral adaptation involving antisocial personality on the one hand, and a
facilitating deviant peer network on the other (Tarter & Vanyukov, 1994;
Wills & Cleary, 1996; Zucker & Ichiyama, 1996). These attributes combined
are more likely to fuel initial alcohol use, as well as the transition into early
problem use.

Until recently, only the adolescent version of these hypotheses has
been tested with some success (Blackson, 1994; Blackson & Tarter, 1994;
Blackson, Tarter, Martin, & Moss, 1994; Wills, Windle & Cleary, 1998). At
this point, a series of prospective studies have established a link between
behavioral undercontrol in early childhood and alcohol dependence in

early adulthood. The first of these studies (Caspi, Moffitt, Newman, & Silva 1996) involves an entire birth cohort of 1,037 children in the Dunedin (New Zealand) Health and Development Study (Silva, 1990), who have been followed since birth, with the most recent outcome data available through early adulthood. Boys rated as undercontrolled (irritable, impulsive, rough, lacking control, and labile in emotional response) were 2.7 times more likely to be diagnosed with alcohol dependence (Caspi et al., 1996). No differences were present between high and low undercontrolled girls. A related series of analyses showed a similar relationship for behavioral inhibition (greater social reticence, fearful and with limited communication, inhibited, upset by strangers), with inhibited boys (but not girls) showing more alcohol-related problems at age 21.

Three other studies have begun with children in middle childhood and early adolescence, thus providing information about developmental variation after preschool. One study using the Swedish Adoption Study database found that child personality patterns at age 11 predicted alcohol abuse/dependence at age 27 (Cloninger, Sigvardsson & Bohman, 1988). Findings indirectly replicate the Dunedin findings, in that both boys who were high in novelty seeking and low in harm avoidance (i.e., behaviorally undercontrolled), as well as those who were high in harm avoidance and low in novelty seeking (i.e., overcontrolled and fearful) were more likely to exhibit alcoholic behaviors at age 27. In a second study, Masse and Tremblay (1997) found teacher ratings at both ages 6 and 10 were predictive of drunkenness onset during the 11–15 year age range. Low fearfulness and hyperactivity were significant predictors of drunkenness onset with the fearfulness indicator working better at age 6 and the hyperactivity indicator working better at age 10.

A third longitudinal study examined aggressive behavior in over 600 subjects followed from age 8 to age 30. It was found that aggression ratings of children by their peers, carried out at age 8, correlated significantly with citation records for Driving While Intoxicated in adulthood ($r = 0.29$, $p < .001$; Eron, Huesmann, Dubow, Romanoff, & Yarmel, 1987).

Taken together, these studies provide major evidence that characteristics from early childhood on are predictive of adult alcohol disorder. However, with the exception of the Masse & Tremblay study (1997), they bypass the onset period altogether. While the mechanism(s) that sustain continuity are not documented, these findings indicate that a substantial amount of the problem behavior syndrome variance noted in middle childhood and adolescence is in place long before middle childhood. The studies also show that there are at least two paths to adult drinking disorder starting with early temperament differences: 1) undercontrol and 2) fearfulness and inhibition. Given the early appearance of these behavioral markers and their consistent identification throughout later childhood, it is likely that some of the behavioral variation is genetically mediated. At the same time, other evidence, discussed below, indicates the importance of socialization effects. Given the robustness of this early display, the findings raise questions about whether preventive intervention beginning in middle childhood will have long-term impact on these high-risk subpopulations.

NEUROBIOLOGICAL EVIDENCE. Deficits in serotonin system output have consistently been linked to both high levels of behavioral aggression and high consumption of alcohol. A large body of evidence indicates that the serotonin system is involved in behavioral regulation, as evidenced by the inverse relationship between impulsive aggression and serotonergic function found both in adult alcoholics and nonalcoholics (e.g., Buydens-Branchey, Branchey, Noumair, & Lieber, 1989; Virkkunen & Linnoila, 1990). Serotonergic status has been indexed by low levels of cerebrospinal fluid (CSF) 5-hydroxyindoleacetic acid (5-HIAA, the major metabolite of serotonin), by downstream measures such as whole blood serotonin (5-HT), and by platelet 5-HT uptake and by density of $5-HT_{2A}$ receptor sites.

Of special interest is the link noted between such deficiencies and the subtype of alcoholism variously known as antisocial alcoholism, or alternately, Type II early onset alcoholism (Fils-Aime et al., 1996). This subtype is distinguished by early onset, strong hereditary likelihood, more severe alcohol-related life problems, and higher levels of violent and aggressive behavior (Babor, 1996). It has been suggested that this early onset subtype has a pre-existing serotonin deficit that manifests both in increased alcohol consumption early in life, as well as poor impulse control (Naranjo et al., 1987). In that regard, it is noteworthy that the appetitive difference has been found to exist even without the antisociality, suggesting that this system operates on a number of different appetitive and expression systems (Fils-Aime et al., 1996). Equally importantly, a small body of literature has noted a parallel relationship among two groups at high risk for later alcoholic disorder: one involving nonalcoholics with a family history positive Ss (LeMarquand, Benkelfat, Pihl, Palmour, & Young, 1999; Rausch, Monteiro, & Schuckit, 1991), the other involving children of alcoholics whose behavioral profile of high behavior problems was indicative of high risk for later alcoholic disorder (Twitchell et al., 1998).

These data suggest that either the same areas of the brain are responsible for both impulsive aggression and a pharmacological reward structure that makes ethanol intake pleasurable, or that different areas of the brain are involved in the same neurochemical architecture. The notion that an appetite for alcohol and/or an enjoyment of its effects, irrespective of a propensity to impulsive and antisocial behavior, is an innate characteristic of the neurochemical architecture of human beings is a relatively novel idea to behavioral scientists. Nonetheless, the serotonin system studies point in that direction.

THE HETEROGENEITY OF INFLUENCES ON ALCOHOL USE DISORDER. Despite these connections, at the behavioral level, the hypothesis that all alcohol problems would be resolved by addressing the problem of antisocial behavior is most likely false. Despite the high association between antisociality and alcohol dependence, only 15% of male and 10% of female alcoholics share this comorbidity. Moreover, the two longest-term child prospective studies with adult outcomes (Caspi et al., 1996; Cloninger et al., 1988) both indicate there is also an overcontrolled and socially inhibited subtype. In addition, anxiety disorders are disproportionately found among persons with alcohol dependence by a ratio of about 2.7:1 (Kessler et al., 1997). Careful inspection of rate differences also shows significant gender-related variation in anxiety subtype. However, it is unclear the extent to which anxiety itself, rather than the specific social inhibition form, is causal. Kushner, Sher, and Breitman (1990) obtained findings consistent with these longitudinal studies in concluding that the primary area of comorbid vulnerability and potential causal mechanism is social phobia. A study done by Schuckit and Hesselbrock (1994), which did not break up the groups in the same manner, is more equivocal.

Depression (characterized in its nonclinical form as negative affectivity) is another specific comorbidity that has been causally linked to the development of alcohol problems and dependence. The odds ratio observed in the National Comorbidity Study (Kessler et al., 1994) for any affective disorder is 3.7:1. Again, there is a significant gender effect; females show an odds ratio of 4.2:1 and males a ratio of 3.2:1 (Kessler et al., 1994). A systematic review of prospective population studies in this area reinforces these strong gender differences and also indicates that in virtually all of them, the depression preceded the alcohol problems/dependence (Wong & Zucker, 2001). The adolescent prospective studies of this relationship also strongly suggest gender variation in this process, with a much stronger relationship observed among girls (Lewinsohn, Hops, Roberts, Seeley, & Andrews, 1993; Windle & Davies, 1999).

Equally important, only 45% of male alcoholics and 55% of female alcoholics have any psychiatric comorbidity (Helzer, Burnam, & McEvoy, 1991). The comorbidity concept is an important one. The National Comorbidity Study (NCS) data (Kessler et al., 1994; Kessler et al., 1997) indicate that diagnostic continuity in adulthood is most likely to be found among that one-sixth of the population who have three or more comorbid disorders, and that, not surprisingly, comorbidity is more likely in those with alcohol dependence rather than abuse. Comorbid anxiety and depression are more common among women, while conduct disorder/antisocial personality disorder is more common among men; and first onset of the alcohol disorder is more often reported to be preceded by the comorbid disorder. Although the order of precedence of symptomatology is retrospective and needs to be regarded with a great deal of caution, these data nonetheless begin to address the issue of what the matrix of onset for later disorder may be, in a manner that is not possible with the large body of adolescent general population studies. They also make the case that the subpopulation of diagnostic significance is small, heavily concentrated, and likely to show continuity over time.

The earlier Epidemiologic Catchment Area data have made this case in a slightly different way. Persons with alcohol abuse/dependence and no co-occurring psychiatric disorder experienced later disorder onset, of lesser severity, and the course of the active diagnosis was shorter than for those with comorbid disorders (Helzer et al., 1991).

In short, there are at least three identifiably different worlds of alcoholic disorder: one of high severity, comorbidity, early onset and longer course; another involving a negative affect pathway, that appears to be more common among females than males; and a third, more transitory group, appearing later, that is much less clearly connected to other forms of misbehavior and symptomatology. Program design, even in adulthood, needs to be different for these phenotypes. The noncomorbid group is more amenable to brief intervention strategies invoking self-education, self-awareness, and self-monitoring procedures as the process by which change is induced (Babor & Grant, 1992; Miller & Munoz, 1976; Miller & Rollnick, 1991; Sanchez-Craig & Wilkinson, 1991). The antisocial group with high comorbidity is most recalcitrant (Babor et al., 1992; Nace, Davis, & Gaspari, 1991; Penick et al., 1994), and requires both longer and more intensive intervention as well as different treatment strategies. Cognitive behavioral intervention rather than interpersonal treatment appears to work better when the alcohol dependence is coupled with antisocial personality disorder, and post-treatment social support appears to worsen outcomes because of the clientele discomfort with social controls (Litt, Babor, Del Boca, Kadden, & Cooney, 1992; Longabaugh et al., 1994). This level of differentiated intervention has not systematically made its way into the prevention armamentarium with youth, although there are some intriguing early attempts in this direction, primarily in family therapy (Szapocznik et al., 1988; Szapocznik, 1996).

A multiple trajectories model has been proposed that takes account of this heterogeneity (Zucker, 2000; Zucker, Fitzgerald, & Moses, 1995). Within the model, onset and rates of development of adolescent alcohol use/problems involve heterogeneous subgroups that have different growth patterns, different patterns of decay, and different social, familial, and biological influencing structures that involve differing contributions of each of these influencing systems. The model specifies that some of these systems are more salient for some subgroups but not others (for example, the serotonergic system in antisocial alcoholism, the ethanol reward system, and possibly the GABA system in nonantisocial alcoholism, the negative affect and dopaminergic systems in negative affect alcoholism). The timing of influence is also different because of the way these systems engage with the normative developmental challenges of different life stages (Zucker, 2000; Zucker, Chermack, & Curran, 2000).

THE RELATIONSHIP BETWEEN ALCOHOL PROBLEMS AND ANTISOCIAL BEHAVIOR.   Despite the heterogeneity of influences on alcohol problems, it is imperative to understand the connections between antisocial behavior and the emergence of alcohol problems.

Considering that (a) the strongest comorbid connection between AUD and other psychiatric disorder is the connection to antisocial personality disorder; (b) antisocial personality disorder, by definition, requires continuation of antisocial behavior, in the form of conduct disorder, from early on in life; and (c) the use of alcohol generally does not begin until late childhood or early adolescence, it is not surprising that the dominant view in the literature is that the direction is causally from antisocial behavior to alcohol problems. The fact that there is also a time-ordered connection between the appearance of the problem behavior syndrome in adolescence and the subsequent development of alcohol use would also appear to support this conclusion.

However, it is unlikely that this relationship is unidirectional. That is, it is unlikely that antisocial behavior simply brings about problem drinking. Other factors influence this relationship and make this unidirectional, univariate model overly simplistic. For example, the correlated nature of the risk structure makes it difficult to disentangle the relationship between antisocial behavior and problem drinking.

There are two reasons for doubting a unidirectional relationship. First, there is a strong comorbid relationship between these two disorders in adulthood. Second, the vast majority of etiologic studies of the development of aggression and conduct disorder do not examine alcohol problems/alcoholism in parents, siblings, and peers as factors that potentially contribute to this association. Thus, it is impossible to model or evaluate the role that alcohol use/alcohol problems has played—either separately or interactively—in mediating this relationship.

With regard to the first point, as already noted, there is substantial evidence that some factors contribute to both syndromes. Insofar as this is correct, the timing of appearance of the two behaviors, although indicating proximal order, may not accurately reflect the shared underlying mechanistic structure. Some of the evidence is neurochemical, while other evidence is neuroanatomical. For example, a substantial body of evidence on the neurocognitive deficits shared by antisocial and alcoholic adults identifies a common pathway of effect from an initially identical set of neurocognitive deficits. The order of relationship is from prefrontal cortical deficits to the behavioral manifestations of attention deficit disorder and other executive function deficits, and then to the emergence of both conduct disorder and substance use disorder (Nigg, 2000; Poon, Ellis, Fitzgerald, & Zucker, 2000). Interestingly, one large national predictive study of child disturbance outcomes over a 3-year interval found that attention problems (a marker of neurocognitive deficits) and delinquent behavior (an indicator of the behavioral undercontrol cluster discussed earlier) were two of the most powerful indicators predicting damaged outcomes in both younger (age 4–11) and older (age 12–16) children (Stanger, Achenbach, & McConaughy, 1993).

With regard to the second point, the order of appearance, to an extent, is a measurement issue. Prior to the overt use of alcohol and other drugs, a cognitive schema needs to be formed which indicates both an awareness of this class of objects, as well as a positive view of their desirability (Zucker, Fitzgerald, & Noll, 1991). Work using both picture tasks and smelling games indicates that the schema structure for alcohol is in place in all populations as early as the age of three. Children already know the rules about use at this age (adults drink, children don't; men drink more than women), and their willingness to assign alcoholic beverage use to hypothetical adults is predicted, even in nursery school, by the consumption levels they observe among their parents (Noll, Zucker, & Greenberg, 1990; Zucker et al., 1995). It remains to be seen whether these rudimentary levels of expectancy will have predictive value in regards to onset of alcohol use and problem use in adolescence. The studies that will test this proposition have not been running long enough to permit this analysis. The point, however, is that the potential is present for such early expectancies to influence behavior in later childhood and adolescence.

A large portion of the etiologic literature on the development of conduct problems indicates that parenting practices are a major mediator of initial child temperament differences, as well as differences at the macro-level, in social disadvantage (Bank, Forgatch, Paterson, & Fetrow, 1993; Deater-Deckard, Dodge, Bates, & Pettit, 1998; Frick et al., 1992). In all of these studies, the parenting is measured, but the level of parental alcohol use—either long-term or short term—and the "wetness" or "dryness" of parents as related to their ability to monitor, provide nurturance, offer effective discipline is not.

The importance of this issue is underscored by the few studies that have relevant information. Two studies (Moos, Finney, & Cronkite, 1990; Puttler, Zucker, Fitzgerald, & Wong, 2001) show that parents in remission have children who are performing better. In particular, the Puttler et al. study focuses more on specific outcome variables related to antisocial behavior—namely level of externalizing behavior and school achievement. These data show that when parents are in remission, externalizing problems are lower and achievement scores are higher.

The Nesting of Risk in High Risk Environments

The fact that the influences on alcohol problems and behavioral problems are correlated can repeatedly be observed. From both etiologic and prevention perspectives, there is special interest in the degree to which risks are correlated, at the individual, familial, and the neighborhood levels. As noted earlier, at the individual level, the literature has increasingly acknowledged the clustering of comorbid symptomatology, social dysfunction, and alcoholism severity among adults (Babor, 1996). In fact, such assortment has been one of the driving forces for the notion that subtypes of disorder need to be demarcated. In the same vein, the association of severe alcoholism with poverty has a long, visible history (Fitzgerald & Zucker, 1995), and recent analyses at the microenvironmental level have documented a clear association between neighborhood disadvantage and alcoholism rates (Zucker, Fitzgerald, Refior, Pallas, & Ellis, 2000). The most common explanation of this has been that poverty, and the neighborhood structure in which it is embedded, drives the alcoholism (i.e., a top-down explanation).

The degree to which individual processes are also at work is less clear. Some evidence suggests that they certainly do come into play—at least for those with the antisocial subtype. For example, antisocial alcoholic men are more likely to marry/couple with antisocial and heavily drinking/alcoholic women (Jester, Zucker, Wong, & Fitzgerald, 2000; Zucker, Ellis, Bingham, & Fitzgerald, 1996), and the families that they create are, therefore, more likely to experience disadvantages in socializing offspring. Antisocial alcoholism is also associated with downward social mobility (Zucker, Ellis, Fitzgerald, Bingham, & Sanford, 1996), and children in these families, even early in life, appear to be developmentally more disadvantaged; that is, they have more learning disabilities and intellectual deficits than do children from families that are alcoholic but not antisocial (Poon et al., 2000; Puttler, Zucker, Fitzgerald, & Bingham, 1998). A risk cumulation theory would suggest that as these factors cumulate; they create an environment that will move the child into peer networks high in aggression, negative mood, and substance use. This, then, will provide a familial, a neighborhood, and peer structure, all of which act in concert to encourage the development of (1) an expectancy structure that is positive toward alcohol and drug use and abuse, (2) very early onset for such use, and (3) a stable repertoire of behaviors that are prototypic for the eventual emergence of abuse/dependence.

It has been suggested that a child's individual risk, when embedded in such enhancing ecological and familial microenvironments, needs to be regarded as a "nesting structure," (Zucker, Fitzgerald et al., 2000) that makes stability of psychopathological outcome much more likely. In other words, a trajectory of development is created that has a consistent outcome because of the coalescence of risk. It has also been argued by Wong, Zucker, Puttler, and Fitzgerald (1999) that this aggregation structure changes the process model of risk. The proximity of a greater number of individual risk factors is more likely to produce overexposure of the risky behavioral repertoire, which, in turn, should create a more rigid high-risk developmental trajectory. The obverse would be anticipated in a less densely risk-laden system. With less risk aggregation, the developmental course should be more open to environmental opportunity, and hence the trajectory should be more fluid.

This line of reasoning is consistent with normative studies of adolescent drug use. Duncan, Duncan, Biglan, and Ary (1998) have shown the cluster of family conflict, association with deviant peers, and poor academic performance has a synergistic effect upon drug use and timing of onset. Also consistent is recent work that shows that most of the association between negative parenting and children's externalizing behavior is explained by environmentally mediated parental effects upon child behavior, rather than on the basis of an evocative gene-environment correlation (O'Connor, Deater-Deckard, Fulker, Rutter, & Plomin, 1998). This aggregated structure offers a challenge for prevention efforts because the cumulative nature of risk makes intervention more difficult in instances when it is needed most (Greenfield & Rogers, 1999; Sinclair & Sillanaukee, 1993).

The Implications of What We Know for Prevention Programming

The evidence presented in this review, as well as by others (Hawkins, Catalano, & Miller, 1992; Hops et al., 1999), indicates that waiting until adolescence to try to prevent alcohol problems may be a mistake, at least for the comorbid problem group. A focused challenge needs to be made to investigators conducting adolescent prevention trials to demonstrate that prevention activity during adolescence is capable of preventing psychiatric disorders in adulthood. Thus far, the longitudinal studies that have begun in early childhood and have continued as far as adulthood indicate that this impact does not occur, at least for those individuals whose functioning is severely compromised as youngsters. By adolescence, some of this population has already been lost to school-based programming, either by refusing such programs or by dropping out early in the intervention process (McCubbin, McCubbin, Thompson, & Han, 1999). Researchers tend not to focus attention on the part of their sample not being reached, partly because there is not much data available on those who refuse intervention, and also because this would tend to undermine their results. Yet this very high-risk subgroup typically ranges from 1/5 to 1/3 of the potential target population, and the clinical literature would suggest that it is with this that greatest comorbidity already exists, and where the greatest likelihood for long-term symptomatic continuity is going to take place (Stark, 1992). On those grounds, it would be worthwhile to encourage the various National Institute of Health organizations who have funded such trials to offer grant supplements to (a) explore the degree to which highest risk young people are lost to the studies and (b) examine the degree to which the interventions being tested are having impact on this subgroup.

An alternative strategy for improving access is to offer prevention programs to adolescents in treatment and juvenile justice settings. Unfortunately, the programming in these settings varies greatly in its attention to the role of the family and other players in the social environment who continue to mediate the ostensive symptomatic stability. In addition, such secondary intervention has already passed the point of origin of the disorders, and reversal of long-term outcomes is likely to be more difficult. A small group of therapists with a family systems focus has shown some success using family therapy alone (Szapocznik, 1996; Szapocznik et al., 1988), as well as combined behavioral and family therapy methods (Waldron, Brody, & Slesnick, 2001) for these very difficult populations.

Nonetheless, the recalcitrance of these youth and the nature of their troubles by the time they arrive in treatment settings, lead to the suggestion that the point of intervention for heavily comorbid adolescents needs to be earlier and followed up with outreach programming. Unfortunately, the cost of such programming, especially if it involves a rigorously population-based design, is one of the most daunting roadblocks to implementation that would address problems of this risk-burdened group. While the recommendation that communities should spend public health or education dollars to implement long-term prevention activity is unrealistic, there are still a number of more viable intervention routes.

One is to shore up Early Head Start/Head Start programs to explicitly reach out to families where informal screening has detected substance abuse in one of the primary caretakers. Another strategy is to gauge child risk by using parent functioning as a marker and point of access to their at-risk children. As shown in Tables 2 and 3, this is a very large population. In the realm of alcohol problems, access could come through mandated family assessment and preventive programming offered as part of a contract whenever parent problems surface. The two most obvious venues for such work are (a) when parents have had trouble with the law (e.g., for drunk driving offenses), and (b) when their alcohol or other drug problems surface in medical settings. Zucker and colleagues have used precisely this strategy in an outreach program for drunk driver fathers (Zucker, Maguin, Noll, Fitzgerald, &, Klinger, 1990; Zucker & Noll, 1987). At the point of conviction and referral for court-mandated substance abuse education, the father was asked if program staff might speak with him and his family. Seventy-nine percent agreed. The family was then offered the opportunity to participate in a program to improve parent-child communications. Seventy-one percent of this group completed at least five sessions, and 57% of those who were offered the program participated for the full 10-month intervention (Maguin, Zucker, & Fitzgerald, 1994). The intervention was successful in reducing child conduct problems and in improving pro-social behavior halfway through the program, at treatment ending, and at a 6-month follow-up (Maguin et al., 1994; Nye, Zucker, & Fitzgerald, 1995, 1999). Luthar and Suchman (2000) provide a parallel example for mothers abusing opiate. The Columbia group found lower maltreatment risk, better child interaction, lower child maladjustment scores, and decreased opiate use in their adjunctive relational/parent practices support program for opiate-abusing mothers.

The fact is that the field has not sufficiently taken advantage of using the parent's problem as an access point for the child, although some literature indicates the presence of cross-generation effects. For example, Kumpfer (1998) reported lower parent drug use as well as decreases in child externalizing behavior from pre- to post-test in the Strengthening Families protocol. Working from a slightly different perspective, O'Farrell and Feehan (1999) noted the major family changes that have been identified as a reliable outcome from behavioral couples therapy. These include reduced family stress, improved marital adjustment, reduced domestic violence and family conflict, reduced risk for separation and divorce, improvement in nurturance and caring, and reduced emotional stress in spouses. They point out that it is an easy and logical next step to the hypothesis that such programs will also have positive effects on children's mental health and social adjustment outcomes. The field has not systematically researched this outcome, although individual programs (e.g., Moos et al., 1990; Puttler et al., 2001) already are confirming this hypothesis.

Families that are at risk for fostering children's alcohol problems can also be identified in medical settings. One avenue is a hospital's emergency department. This unit sees a high number of alcoholic and alcohol-abusing adults, and, with the proper approach, their families are potentially accessible. Recent work has also identified these settings as high-density pass-through points for other alcohol-related risk factors such as spousal abuse (Melnick et al., 2000) and adolescent drinking (Barnett et al., 1998). Pediatric emergency departments also offer a high-density access point, given that lower income households who do not have access to managed care use these facilities for both regular medical care (e.g., a child with the flu) as well as emergencies pertaining to risky behavior of themselves and their children (for example, cuts, broken limbs, or problem drinking difficulties, including DUIL; Barnett, Monti, & Wood, 2001; Cunningham, personal communication, February 2000).

To take this one step further, the development of family assessment and treatment modules that become integrated parts of parent treatment contracts is not only feasible for situations involving behavioral disorders, but also at times of contact for medical care in primary health care settings (Blow, Greden, Neal, & Carli, 2000). This should be a reachable goal, and it has the potential to provide a solution to the problem of prevention/intervention cost. Thus, a potential national agenda would be to lobby for add-on components to existing adult treatments that would address child problems that are already being documented in the system, but have not yet reached public view. In addition, the prevention community needs to move beyond demonstration projects and into the clinical trial phase in order to test for savings to the health care/managed care system and future generations of children.

Conclusion

Efforts to prevent alcohol-related problems need to be informed by an understanding of the special nature of alcohol in our society. Alcohol use contributes to many problems in our society, including alcohol-related auto accidents, delinquency, and poorer school performance. Yet, alcohol use is also a central feature of many important cultural activities and, when used in moderation, may have benefits for cardiovascular functioning. There are a variety of inter-connected factors contributing to the development of alcohol problems. A particularly important one is behavioral undercontrol and associated patterns of aggressive behavior, since the subgroup of young people who have both alcohol and aggressive behavior problems are particularly prone to serious and continued problems in adulthood. It is unlikely that the prevention of these problems can be achieved solely through interventions delivered in adolescence, and prevention programs targeting this age group need to evaluate whether they prevent alcohol abuse and other problems in adulthood. Interventions targeting families that are at high risk for raising children with aggressive behavior and alcohol problems could be targeted through preventive programs that reach them through the justice system or the medical care system. It may also be possible to prevent these problems through programs that reach at-risk children as early as preschool.

References

Ary, D.V., Tildesley, E., Hops, H., & Andrews, J. (1993). The influence of parent, sibling, and peer modeling and attitudes on adolescent use of alcohol. *International Journal of the Addictions, 28*, 853–80.

Andrews, J.A., Hops, H., & Duncan, S.C. (1997). Adolescent modeling of parent substance use: The moderating effect of the relationship with the parent. *Journal of Family Psychology, 11*, 259–70.

Babor, T.F. (1996). The classification of alcoholics: Typology theories from the 19th century to the present. *Alcohol Health and Research World, 20*, 6–17.

Babor, T.F., Dolinsky, Z.S., Meyer, R.E., Hesselbrock, M., Hofman, M., & Tennen, H. (1992). Types of alcoholics: Concurrent and predictive validity of some common classification schemes. *British Journal of Addictions, 87*, 1415–31.

Babor, T.F., & Grant, M. (1992). (Eds). *Programme on substance abuse: Project on identification and management of alcohol related problems. Report on Phase II: A randomized clinical trial of brief interventions in primary health care.* New York: World Health Organization.

Bachman, J.G., Wadsworth, K.N., O'Malley, P.M., Johnston, L.D., & Schulenberg, J.E. (1997). *Smoking, drinking and drug use in young adulthood: The impact of new freedoms and new responsibilities.* Mahwah, NJ: Lawrence Erlbaum.

Bank, L., Forgatch, M.S., Paterson, G.R., & Fetrow, R.A. (1993). Parenting practices of single mothers: Mediators of negative contextual factors. *Journal of Marriage and the Family, 55*, 371–84.

Barnett, N.P., Monti, P.M., & Wood, M.D. (2001). Motivational interviewing for alcohol-involved adolescents in the emergency room. In E.F. Wagner & H.B. Waldron (Eds.), *Innovations in adolescent substance abuse intervention* (pp. 232–57). NYC: Elsevier.

Barnett, N.P., Spirito, A., Colby, S.M., Vallee, J.A., Woolard, R., Lewander, W., et al. (1998). Detection of alcohol use in adolescent patients in the emergency department. *Academic Emergency Medicine, 5*, 607–12.

Blackson, T. (1994). Temperament: A salient correlate of risk factors for drug abuse. *Drug and Alcohol Dependence, 36*, 205–14.

Blackson, T.C., & Tarter, R.E. (1994). Individual, family, and peer affiliation factors predisposing to early-age onset of alcohol and drug use. *Alcoholism: Clinical and Experimental Research, 18*, 813–21.

Blackson, T.C., Tarter, R.E., Martin, R.E., & Moss, H.B. (1994). Temperament-induced father-son family dysfunction: Etiologic implications for child behavior problems and substance abuse. *American Journal of Orthopsychiatry, 62*, 280–92.

Blanton, H., Gibbons, F.X., Gerrard, M., Conger, K.J., & Smith, G.E. (1997). Role of family and peers in the development of prototypes associated with substance use. *Journal of Family Psychology, 11,* 271–88.

Blow, F.C., Greden, J.F., Neal, D., & Carli, T. (2000). *Evaluation program for the Washtenaw Integrated Project.* Unpublished grant proposal, University of Michigan, Department of Psychiatry.

Buydens-Branchey, L., Branchey, M.H., Noumair, D., & Lieber, C.S. (1989). Age of alcoholism onset. II. Relationship to susceptibility to serotonin precursor availability. *Archives of General Psychiatry, 46,* 231–36.

Caspi, A., Moffitt, T.E., Newman, D.L., & Silva, E.A. (1996). Behavioral observations at age 3 years predict adult psychiatric disorders: Longitudinal evidence from a birth cohort. *Archives of General Psychiatry, 53,* 1033–39.

Cloninger, C.R., Sigvardsson, S., & Bohman, M. (1988). Childhood personality predicts alcohol abuse in young adults. *Alcoholism: Clinical and Experimental Research, 12,* 494–505.

Deater-Deckard, K., Dodge, K.A., Bates, J.A., & Pettit, G.S. (1998). Multiple risk factors in the development of externalizing behavior problems: Group and individual differences. *Development & Psychopathology, 10,* 469–93.

Dishion, T.J., & Loeber, R. (1985). Adolescent marijuana and alcohol use: The role of parents and peers revisited. *American Journal of Drug and Alcohol Abuse, 11,* 11–25.

Dishion, T.J., Patterson, G.R., & Reid, J.R. (1988). Parent and peer factors associated with drug sampling in early adolescence: Implications for treatment. *NIDA Research Monograph, 77,* 69–93.

Donaldson, S.I., Graham, J.W., & Hansen, W.B. (1995). Resistance-skills training and onset of alcohol use: Evidence for beneficial and potentially harmful effects in public schools and in private Catholic schools. *Health Psychology, 14,* 291–300.

Donovan, J.E., & Jessor, R. (1985). Structure of problem behavior in adolescence and young adulthood. *Journal of Consulting and Clinical Psychology, 53,* 890–904.

Duncan, S.C., Duncan, T.E., Biglan, A., & Ary, D. (1998). Contributions of the social context to the development of adolescent substance use: A multivariate latent growth modeling approach. *Drug and Alcohol Dependence, 50,* 57–71.

Eron, L.D., Huesmann, L.R., Dubow, E., Romanoff, R., & Yarmel, P.W. (1987). Aggression and its correlates over 22 years. In D.H. Crowell, I.M. Evans, & C.R. O'Donnell (Eds.), *Childhood aggression and violence* (pp. 249–262). New York: Plenum.

Fils-Aime, M., Eckardt, M., George, D., Brown, G., Mefford, I., & Linnoila, M. (1996). Early-onset alcoholics have lower CSF 5-HIAA than late-onset alcoholics. *Archives of General Psychiatry 53,* 211–16.

Fitzgerald, H.E., & Zucker, R.A. (1995). Socioeconomic status and alcoholism: Structuring developmental pathways to addiction. In H.E. Fitzgerald, B.M. Lester, & B. Zuckerman (Eds.), *Children of poverty* (pp. 125–47). New York: Garland Press.

Frick, P.J., Leahy, B.B., Loeber, R., Stouthamer-Loeber, M., Christ, M.A.G., & Hanson, K. (1992). Familial risk factors to oppositional defiant disorder and conduct disorder: Parent psychopathology and maternal parenting. *Journal of Consulting and Clinical Psychology, 60,* 49–55.

Garg, R., Wagener, D.K., & Madens, J.H. (1993). Alcohol consumption and risk of ischemic heart disease in women. *Archives of Internal Medicine, 153,* 1211–16.

Grant, B.F. (1997). Prevalence and correlates of alcohol use and DSM-IV alcohol dependence in the United States: Results of the national longitudinal alcohol epidemiologic survey. *Journal of Studies on Alcohol, 58,* 464–73.

Greenfield, T.K., & Rogers, J.D. (1999). Who drinks most of the alcohol in the U.S.? The policy implications. *Journal of Studies on Alcohol, 60,* 78–89.

Hansen, W. (1988). Theory and implementation of the social influence model of primary prevention. In *Office for Substance Abuse Prevention Monograph No. 3: Prevention research findings: 1988* (DHHS Publication No. ADM 88-1615, pp. 93–107). Washington, DC: Government Printing Office.

Hawkins, J.D., Catalano, R.F., & Miller, J.Y. (1992). Risk and protective factors for alcohol and other drug problems in adolescence and early adulthood: Implications for substance abuse prevention. *Psychological Bulletin, 112*, 64–105.

Helzer, J.E., Burnam, A., & McEvoy, L.T. (1991). Alcohol abuse and dependence. In L.H. Robins & D.A. Regier (Eds.), *Psychiatric disorders in America* (pp. 81–115). NYC: Free Press.

Hops, H., Davis, E.B., & Lewin, L.M. (1999). The development of alcohol and other substance use: A gender study of family and peer context. *Journal of Studies on Alcohol Supplement, 13*, 22–31.

Huang, L.X., Cerbone, F.G., & Gfroerer, J.C. (1998). Children at risk because of substance abuse. In Office of Applied Studies, Substance Abuse and Mental Health Services Administration (Ed.), *Analyses of substance abuse and treatment need issues* (DHHS Publication No. SMA 98-3227, pp. 5–18). Rockville, MD: Author.

Jacob, T., & Leonard, K. (1994). Family and peer influences in the development of adolescent alcohol abuse. In R. Zucker, G. Boyd, & J. Howard (Eds.), *Development of alcohol problems: Exploring the biopsychosocial matrix of risk. NIAAA Research Monograph No. 26* (pp. 123–55). Rockville, MD: National Institute on Alcohol Abuse & Alcoholism.

Jessor, R., Costa, F., Jessor, L., & Donovan, J.E. (1983) Time of first intercourse: A prospective study. *Journal of Personality and Social Psychology, 44*, 608–26.

Jessor, R., Donovan, J.E., & Costa, F.M. (1991). *Beyond adolescence: Problem behavior and young adult development.* Cambridge, England: Cambridge University Press.

Jessor, R., & Jessor, S.L. (1977). *Problem behavior and psychosocial development: A longitudinal study of youth.* New York: Academic Press.

Jessor, S.L., & Jessor, R. (1975). Transition from virginity to non-virginity among youth: A social-psychological study over time. *Developmental Psychology, 11*, 473–84.

Jester, J.M., Zucker, R.A., Wong, M.M., & Fitzgerald, H.E. (2000). Marital assortment in high-risk population [Abstract]. *Alcoholism: Clinical and Experimental Research, 24*, 36A.

Johnston, L.D., O'Malley, P.M., & Bachman, J.G. (1997). *National survey results on drug use from the Monitoring The Future study, 1975–1995: Vol. 1: Secondary school students.* Rockville, MD: National Institute on Drug Abuse.

Kandel, D.B. (Ed.). (1978). *Longitudinal research on drug use: Empirical findings and methodological issues.* Washington, DC: Hemisphere Publishing.

Kessler, R.C., Crum, R.M., Warner, L.A., Nelson, C.B., Schulenberg, J., & Anthony, J.C. (1997). Lifetime co-occurrence of DSM-III-R alcohol abuse and dependence with other psychiatric disorders in the National Comorbidity Study. *Archives of General Psychiatry, 54*, 313–21.

Kessler, R.C., McGonagle, K.A., Zhao, S., Nelson, C.B., Hughs, M., Eshleman, S., Wittchen, H.U., & Kendler, K.S. (1994). Lifetime and 12-month prevalence of DSM-III-R psychiatric disorders in the United States. *Archives of General Psychiatry, 51*, 8–19.

Klatsky, A.L. (1994). Epidemiology of coronary heart disease—Influence of alcohol. *Alcoholism: Clinical and Experimental Research, 18*, 88–96.

Klein, H. (1991). Cultural determinants of alcohol use in the United States. In D.J. Pittman & H.R. White (Eds.), *Society, culture, and drinking patterns reexamined* (pp. 114–34). New Brunswick, NJ: Rutgers Center of Alcohol Studies.

Kumpfer, K. (1998). Selective preventive interventions: The Strengthening Families program. In R.S. Ashery, E.B. Robertson, & K.L. Kumpfer (Eds.), *Drug abuse prevention through family interventions. NIDA Monograph 177* (pp. 160–207). Rockville, MD: National Institute on Drug Abuse.

Kushner, M., Sher, K.J., & Breitman, B. (1990). The relation between alcohol problems and the anxiety disorders. *American Journal of Psychiatry, 147*, 685–95.

LeMarquand, D.G., Benkelfat, C., Pihl, R.O., Palmour, R.M., & Young, S.N. (1999). Behavioral disinhibition induced by tryptophan depletion in nonalcoholic young men with multigenerational family histories of paternal alcoholism. *American Journal of Psychiatry, 156*, 1771–79.

Lewinsohn, P.M., Hops, H., Roberts, R.E., Seeley, J.R., & Andrews, J.A. (1993). Adolescent psychopathology: I. Prevalence and incidence of depression and other DSM-III-R disorders in high school students. *Journal of Abnormal Psychology, 102*, 133–44.

Litt, M.D., Babor, T.F., Del Boca, F.K., Kadden, R.M., & Cooney, N.L. (1992). Types of alcoholics: II. Application of an empirically derived typology to treatment matching. *Archives of General Psychiatry, 49*, 609–14.

Longabaugh, R., Rubin, A., Malloy, P., Beattie, M., Clifford, P.R., & Noel, N. (1994). Drinking outcomes of alcohol abusers diagnosed as antisocial personality disorder. *Alcoholism: Clinical and Experimental Research, 18*, 778–85.

Luthar, S.S., & Suchman, N.E. (2000). Relational psychotherapy mothers' group: A developmentally informed intervention for at-risk mothers. *Development and Psychopathology, 12*, 235–53.

MacKinnon, D.P., Johnson, C.A., Pentz, M.A., Dwyer, J.H., Hansen, W.B., Flay, B.R., & Wang, E.Y. (1991). Mediating mechanisms in a school-based drug prevention program: first-year effects of the Midwestern Prevention Project. *Health Psychology, 10*, 164–72.

Maddox, G.L., & McCall, B.C. (1964). *Drinking among teenagers.* New Brunswick, NJ: Rutgers Center of Alcohol Studies.

Maggs, J.L. (1997). Alcohol use and binge drinking as goal-directed action during the transition to post-secondary education. In J. Schulenberg, J.L. Maggs, & K. Hurrelmann (Eds.), *Health risks & developmental transitions during adolescence* (pp. 345–71). NY: Cambridge University Press.

Maguin, E., Zucker, R.A., & Fitzgerald, H.E. (1994). The path to alcohol problems through conduct problems: A family based approach to very early intervention with risk. *Journal of Research on Adolescence, 4*, 249–69.

Masse, L.C., & Tremblay, R.E. (1997). Behavior of boys in kindergarten and the onset of substance use during adolescence. *Archives of General Psychiatry, 54*, 62–68.

McCubbin, H.I., McCubbin, M.A., Thompson, A.I. & Han, S.Y. (1999). Contextualizing family risk factors for alcoholism and alcohol abuse. *Journal of Studies on Alcohol Supplement, 13*, 75–78.

Melnick, D.M., Maio, R.F., Blow, F.C., Wang, S.C., Pomerantz, R., Kane, M.L., et al. (2000, October). *Preliminary results of screening female trauma inpatients for a history of domestic violence and alcohol abuse* [Abstract]. Paper presented at the Frederick A. Coller Surgical Society meeting, Ann Arbor, MI.

Miller, G.J., Beckles, G.L., Maude, G.H., & Carson, D.C. (1990). Alcohol consumption: Protection against coronary heart disease and risks to health. *International Journal of Epidemiology, 19*, 923–30.

Miller, W.R., & Munoz, R.F. (1976). *How to control your drinking.* Englewood Cliffs, NJ: Prentice-Hall.

Miller, W.R., & Rollnick, S. (1991). *Motivational interviewing: Preparing people to change addictive behavior.* New York: Guilford Press.

Moos, R.H., Finney, J.W., & Cronkite, R.C. (1990). *Alcoholism treatment: Context, process, and outcome.* New York: Oxford University Press.

58 Robert A. Zucker

Nace, E.P., Davis, C.W., & Gaspari, J.P. (1991). Axis II comorbidity in substance abusers. *American Journal of Psychiatry, 148,* 118–20.

Naranjo, C.A., Sellers, E.M., Sullivan, J.T., Woodley, D., Kadlec, K., & Sykora, K. (1987). The serotonin uptake inhibitor citalopram attenuates ethanol intake. *Clinical Pharmacology and Therapeutics, 41,* 266–274.

Nigg, J.T. (2000). On inhibition/disinhibition in developmental psychopathology: Views from cognitive and personality psychology and a working inhibition taxonomy. *Psychological Bulletin, 126,* 220–46.

Noll, R.B., Zucker, R.A., & Greenberg, G.S. (1990). Identification of alcohol by smell among preschoolers: Evidence for early socialization about drugs occurring in the home. *Child Development, 61,* 1520–27.

Nye, C.L., Zucker, R.A., & Fitzgerald, H.E. (1995). Early intervention in the path to alcohol problems through conduct problems: Treatment involvement and child behavior change. *Journal of Consulting and Clinical Psychology, 63,* 831–40.

Nye, C.L., Zucker, R.A., & Fitzgerald, H.E. (1999). Early family-based intervention in the path to alcohol problems: Rationale and relationship between treatment process characteristics and child and parenting outcomes. *Journal of Studies on Alcohol Supplement, 13,* 10–21.

O'Farrell, T J., & Feehan, M. (1999). Alcoholism treatment and the family: Do family and individual treatments for alcoholic adults have preventive effects for children. *Journal of Studies on Alcohol Supplement, 13,* 125–29.

O'Connor, T.G., Deater-Deckard, K., Fulker, D., Rutter, M., & Plomin, R. (1998). Genotype-environment correlations in late childhood and early adolescence: Antisocial behavior problems and coercive parenting. *Developmental Psychology, 34,* 970–81.

Penick, E.C., Powell, B.J., Nickel, E.J., Bingham, S.F., Riesenmy, K.R., Read, M.R., et al. (1994). Comorbidity of lifetime psychiatric disorder among male alcoholic patients. *Alcoholism: Clinical and Experimental Research, 18,* 1289–93.

Perry, C.L., & Jessor, R. (1985). The concept of health promotion and the prevention of adolescent drug use. *Health Education Quarterly, 12,* 169–84.

Perry, C.L., Williams, C.L., Veblen-Mortenson, S., Toomey, T.L., Komro, K.A., Anstine, P.S., et al. (1996). Project Northland: Outcomes of a community wide alcohol use prevention program during early adolescence. *American Journal of Public Health, 86,* 956–65.

Poon, E., Ellis, D.A., Fitzgerald, H.E., & Zucker, R.A. (2000). Intellectual, cognitive and academic performances among sons of alcoholics during the early elementary school years: Differences related to subtypes of familial alcoholism. *Alcoholism: Clinical and Experimental Research, 24,* 1020–27.

Puttler, L.I., Zucker, R.A., Fitzgerald, H.E., & Bingham, C.R. (1998). Behavioral outcomes among children of alcoholics during the early and middle childhood years: Familial subtype variations. *Alcoholism: Clinical and Experimental Research, 22,* 1962–72.

Puttler, L.I., Zucker, R.A., & Fitzgerald, H.E., & Wong, M.E. (2001). *Outcome differences among children of alcoholics during early and middle childhood as a function of change in paternal recovery status.* Manuscript submitted for publication.

Rausch, J.L., Monteiro, M.G., & Schuckit, M.A. (1991). Platelet serotonin uptake in men with family histories of alcoholism. *Neuropsychopharmacology, 4,* 83–86.

Regier, D.A., Farmer, M.E., Rae, D.S., Locke, B.Z., Keith, S.J., Judd, L.L., et al. (1990). Comorbidity of mental disorders with alcohol and other drug abuse. *Journal of the American Medical Association, 19,* 2511–18.

Sanchez-Craig, M., & Wilkinson, D.A. (1991). Brief interventions for alcohol and drug dependence: What makes them work. In J. White, R. Ali, & P. Christie (Eds.), *Drug problems in society: Dimensions and perspective.* Parkside, South Australia: Drug and Alcohol Service Council.

Schuckit, M., & Hesselbrock, V.M. (1994). Alcohol dependence and anxiety disorders: What is the relationship? *American Journal of Psychiatry, 151*, 1723–34.

Schulenberg, J.E., & Maggs, J.L. (2002). A developmental perspective on alcohol use and heavy drinking during adolescence and the transition to young adulthood. *Journal of Studies on Alcohol Supplement, 14*, 54–70.

Schulenberg, J., Maggs, J.L., Long, S.W., Sher, K.J., Gotham, H.J., Baer, J.S., Kivlahan, D.R., Marlatt, G.A., & Zucker, R.A. (2001). The problem of college drinking: Insights from a developmental perspective. *Alcoholism: Clinical & Experimental Research, 25*, 473–77.

Schulenberg, J., Maggs, J.L., Steinman, K., & Zucker, R.A. (2001). Development matters: Taking the long view on substance abuse etiology and intervention during adolescence. In P.M. Monti, S.M. Colby, & T.A. O'Leary (Eds.), *Adolescents, alcohol, and substance abuse: Reaching teens through brief intervention* (pp. 19–57). New York: Guilford Press.

Schulenberg, J., O'Malley, P.M., Bachman, J.G., Wadsworth, K.N., & Johnston, L.D. (1996). Getting drunk and growing up: Trajectories of frequent binge drinking during the transition to early adulthood. *Journal of Studies on Alcohol, 57*, 289–304.

Schulenberg, J., Wadsworth, K.N., O'Malley, P.M., Bachman, J.G., & Johnston, L.D. (1996). Adolescent risk factors for binge drinking during the transition to young adulthood: Variable- and pattern-centered approaches to change. *Developmental Psychology, 32*, 659–74.

Silva, P.A. (1990). The Dunedin Multidisciplinary Health and Development study: A 15-year longitudinal study. *Pediatric and Perinatal Epidemiology, 4*, 96–127.

Sinclair, J.D., & Sillanaukee, P. (1993). Comments on "The preventive paradox: A critical examination." *Addiction, 88*, 591–95.

Stanger, C., Achenbach, T.M., & McConaughy, S.M. (1993). Three-year course of behavioral/emotional problems in a national sample of 4- to 16-year olds: 3. Predictors of signs of disturbance. *Journal of Consulting and Clinical Psychology, 61*, 839–48.

Stark, M.J. (1992). Dropping out of substance abuse treatment: A clinically oriented review. *Clinical Psychology Review, 12*, 93–116.

Substance Abuse and Mental Health Services Administration (SAMHSA). (1996). *National Household Survey on Drug Abuse: Population Estimates, 1995.* DHHS Pub. No. SMA 96-3095. Washington, DC: Supt. of Docs, U.S. Government Printing Office

Substance Abuse and Mental Health Services Administration (SAMHSA), Office of Applied Studies. (1998). *Preliminary results from the 1997 National Household Survey on Drug Abuse.* DHHS Pub. No. SMA 98-3251. Rockville, MD: Author.

Szapocznik, J. (1996, January). *Scientific findings that have emerged from family intervention research at the Spanish Family Guidance Center and the Center for Family Studies.* Paper presented at the NIDA Technical Review on Drug Abuse Prevention Through Family Interventions, Gaithersburg, MD.

Szapocznik, J., Perez-Vidal, A., Brickman, A.L., Foote, F.H., Santestaban, D., Hervis, O., et al. (1988). Engaging adolescent drug abusers and their families in treatment: A strategic structural systems approach. *Journal of Consulting and Clinical Psychology, 56*, 552–57.

Tarter, R.E., & Vanyukov, M.M. (1994). Stepwise developmental model of alcoholism etiology. In R.A. Zucker, J. Howard, & G.M. Boyd (Eds.), *The development of alcohol problems: Exploring the biopsychosocial matrix of risk. NIAAA research monograph No. 26* (pp. 303–30). Rockville, MD: U.S. Department of Health and Human Services.

Twitchell, G.R., Hanna, G.L., Cook, E.H., Fitzgerald, H.E., Zucker, R.A., & Little, K.Y. (1998). Overt behavior problems and serotonergic function in middle childhood among male and female offspring of alcoholic fathers. *Alcoholism: Clinical and Experimental Research, 22*, 1340–48.

Virkkunen, M., & Linnoila, M. (1990). Serotonin in early onset, male alcoholics with violent behavior. *Annals of Medicine, 22*, 327–31.

Wagenaar, A.C., & Perry, C.L. (1995). Community strategies for the reduction of youth drinking: Theory and application. In G.M. Boyd (Ed.), *Alcohol problems among adolescents: Current directions in prevention research* (pp. 197–223). Hillsdale, NJ: Lawrence Erlbaum.

Waldron, H.B., Brody, J.L., & Slesnick, N. (2001). Integrative behavioral and family therapy for adolescent substance abuse. In P.M. Monti, S.M. Colby, & T.A. O'Leary (Eds.), *Adolescents, alcohol, and substance abuse: Reaching teens through brief intervention* (pp. 216–43). New York: Guilford Press.

Weber, M.D., Graham, J.W., Hansen, W.B., Flay, R.B., & Anderson, C.A. (1989). Evidence for two paths of alcohol use onset in adolescents. *Addictive Behaviors, 14*, 399–408.

Williams, C.L., Perry, C.L., Farbakhsh, K., & Veblen-Mortenson, S. (1999). Project Northland: Comprehensive alcohol use prevention for young adolescents, their parents, schools, peers and communities. *Journal of Studies on Alcohol Supplement, 13*, 112–24.

Wills, T.A., & Cleary, S.C. (1996). How are social support effects mediated? A test with parental support and adolescent substance use. *Journal of Personality and Social Psychology, 71*, 937–52.

Wills, T.A., Windle, M., & Cleary, S.D. (1998). Temperament and novelty-seeking in adolescent substance use: Convergence of dimensions of temperament with constructs from Cloninger's theory. *Journal of Personality and Social Psychology, 74*, 387–406.

Windle, M., & Davies, P.T. (1999). Depression and heavy alcohol use among adolescents: Concurrent and prospective relations. *Development and Psychopathology, 11*, 823–44.

Wong, M.M., & Zucker, R.A. (2001). *The relationship of depression to alcohol problems: A review.* Manuscript submitted for publication.

Wong, M.M., Zucker, R.A., Puttler, L.I., & Fitzgerald, H.E. (1999). Heterogeneity of risk aggregation for alcohol problems between early and middle childhood: Nesting structure variations. *Development and Psychopathology, 11*, 727–44.

Wynn, S.R., Schulenberg, J., Maggs, J.E., & Zucker, R.A. (2000). Preventing alcohol misuse: The impact of refusal skills and norms. *Psychology of Addictive Behaviors, 14*, 36–47.

Zucker, R.A. (2000). Alcohol involvement over the life course. In: National Institute on Alcohol Abuse and Alcoholism (Ed.), *Tenth Special Report to the U.S. Congress on Alcohol and Health (AH10)* (pp. 28–53). Rockville, MD: NIAA.

Zucker, R.A., Chermack, S.T., & Curran, G.M. (2000) Alcoholism: A lifespan perspective on etiology and course. In A.J. Sameroff, M. Lewis & S. Miller (Eds.), *Handbook of Developmental Psychopathology* (2nd ed.) (pp. 569–87) New York: Plenum.

Zucker, R.A., Ellis, D.A., Bingham, C.R., & Fitzgerald, H.E. (1996). The development of alcoholic subtypes: Risk variation among alcoholic families during the early childhood years. *Alcohol Health and Research World, 20*, 46–54.

Zucker, R.A., Ellis, D.A., Fitzgerald, H.E., Bingham, C.R., & Sanford, K.P. (1996). Other evidence for at least two alcoholisms, II: Life course variation in antisociality and heterogeneity of alcoholic outcome. *Development and Psychopathology, 8*, 831–48.

Zucker, R.A., Fitzgerald, H.E., & Moses, H.D. (1995) Emergence of alcohol problems and several alcoholisms: A developmental perspective on etiologic theory and life course trajectory. In D. Cicchetti & D.J. Cohen (Eds.), *Developmental psychopathology, volume 2: Risk, disorder, and adaptation* (pp. 677–711). New York: Wiley & Son.

Zucker, R.A., Fitzgerald, H.E., & Noll, R.B. (1991, April). The development of cognitive schemas about drugs among preschoolers. In: *The socialization of drinking in children.* Symposium conducted at the meeting of the Society for Research in Child Development, Seattle, WA.

Zucker, R.A., Fitzgerald, H.E., Refior, S.K., Pallas, D.M., & Ellis, D.A. (In press). The clinical and social ecology of childhood for children of alcoholics: Description and implications for a differentiated social policy. In: H.E. Fitzgerald, B.M. Lester & B.S. Zuckerman (Eds.) *Children of addiction*. New York: Garland Press.

Zucker, R.A., & Ichiyama, M.A. (1996). Self-regulation theory: A model of etiology or a route into changing troubled human behavior? *Psychological Inquiry, 7*, 85–89.

Zucker, R.A., Maguin, E.T., Noll, R.B., Fitzgerald, H.E., & Klinger, M.T. (1990, August). *A prevention program for preschool COAs Design and early effects*. Paper presented at the American Psychological Association Meeting, Boston, MA

Zucker, R.A., & Noll, R.B. (1987). The interaction of child and environment in the early development of drug involvement: A far ranging review and a planned very early intervention. *Drugs and Society, 2*, 57–97.

Chapter 3

The Prevention of Tobacco Use

Anthony Biglan and Herbert H. Severson

Cigarette smoking is the number one preventable cause of disease and death in the United States. Smoking is a firmly established cause of numerous cancers, heart disease, emphysema, and pulmonary diseases. Smoking is the main cause of 87% of deaths from lung cancer, 30% of all cancer deaths, 82% of all deaths from pulmonary disease, and 21% of death from chronic heart disease (Centers for Disease Control and Prevention [CDC], 1989). For the population, this results in premature mortality that translates into 6 million years of life lost each year (*Smoking Related Deaths*, 1993). The Office of Technology Assessment put the cost of smoking at $68 billion with $20.8 billion in health care costs and the rest due to lost productivity due to disability or premature death (*Smoking Related Deaths*, 1993). Indeed, it is the number one preventable cause of disease and death (CDC, 1990). Although most of the health consequences of smoking and smokeless tobacco use occur long after adolescence, most smokers become addicted during adolescence (U.S. Department of Health and Human Services [USDHHS], 1994) and it is estimated that a third of adolescents who begin smoking will eventually die of a smoking-related illness. For these reasons, the prevention of youthful tobacco use has become a major priority for public health.

Some health consequences of smoking in adolescence are detectable, including increased respiratory infections and lessened lung capacity (USDHHS, 1994). However, the size and seriousness of these effects are probably too small, by themselves, to justify giving priority to smoking prevention. There is also the problem of teenage girls becoming pregnant and smoking during their pregnancy. The deleterious consequences of maternal smoking include low birth weight, pre-term delivery, spontaneous

63

abortion, and perinatal death, including Sudden Infant Death Syndrome (SIDS; Lightwood, Phibbs, & Glantz, 1999; Lowe, Balanda, & Clare, 1998).

Smokeless tobacco (SLT) use is a related and growing public health problem. While the per capita consumption of cigarettes has declined in the United States, there has been an increase in the use of moist snuff and chewing tobacco, especially by young males. This behavior occurs almost entirely among boys and it is pervasive only in certain regions of the country, e.g., the South and the West (USDHHS, 1994). Smokeless tobacco or "spit tobacco" (the term preferred by the public health community to denote its filthy nature) contains several clearly established carcinogens (USDHHS, 1989). The regular use of SLT causes periodontal disease, oral lesions, and oral cancer (USDHHS, 1989). Moreover, teens using SLT are more likely to become regular smokers (Ary, Lichtenstein, & Severson, 1987; Severson, Lichtenstein, & Gallison, 1985). This is likely due to the adolescent developing an addiction to nicotine and switching to cigarettes when he encounters social pressures not to chew or dip.

The Assessment of Adolescent Smoking Behavior

Adolescent smoking has been defined variously in terms of self-reported smoking in the last week or the last month. There is not clear agreement about which of these is a "better" measure. Typically, the Centers for Disease Control and Prevention's Youth Risk Behavior Survey, as well as in-state reports, have focused on the prevalence of smoking in the last month.

From the standpoint of achieving a reliable measure of smoking, there are well-established advantages to creating a composite index from a number of questionnaire items. For example, Biglan, Ary, Smolkowski, Duncan, and Black (2000) composed an index of weekly smoking based on answers to questions about smoking in the last day, week, and month. They also asked the respondent to indicate level of smoking, with ten choices ranging from "never smoked, not even a puff" to "a few times each month" to "a pack or more each day."

There is some research on the validity of adolescent self-reports of smoking. Researchers have attempted to validate self-report by comparing it to expired-air carbon monoxide and saliva thiocyanate measures (e.g., Biglan, Gallison, Ary, & Thompson, 1985; Pechacek et al., 1984). In general, these measures do correlate with self-report measures. For example, Biglan et al. (1985) found that expired-air carbon monoxide correlated .71 with an index of weekly smoking. In addition, the effects of anonymity and the collection of biochemical measures on self-reporting have been investigated. In general, when adolescents are told that the biochemical measures that are being collected will be used to determine who smokes, the proportion of respondents who self-report smoking increases (Murray, O'Connell, Schmid, & Perry, 1987). Similarly, anonymity increases the level of self-report (Murray & Perry, 1987). However, neither of these effects is very large and it is unlikely that they have much effect on the validity of self-report measures of smoking when they are used to assess the effects of interventions or, more generally, changes in smoking prevalence, because all respondents are providing their responses under the same conditions.

The Assessment of Smokeless Tobacco

The use of smokeless tobacco in the form of chewing tobacco and moist snuff has been measured in a way parallel to that for smoking. The usual items assessing use among adolescents are whether there has been any use in the past seven days or any use in the past 30 days. Assessment of SLT presents some unique challenges in that there is no single dose standardized like a single cigarette and the amount of tobacco used in a single dip or chew can vary considerably. Additionally, the time one keeps the dip in the mouth may vary from a few minutes to an hour. The most useful items to assess total use of SLT have included queries like "how many days does a tin last," "how many dips per day," and "how long do you keep a dip or chew in your mouth before taking another dip?" There is a high inter-correlation among these self-report items; plus, they correlate moderately well with biochemical verification using saliva cotinine (Severson, Eakin, Lichtenstein, & Stevens, 1990).

The Prevalence of Adolescent Smoking

Table 1 presents the monthly prevalence of smoking among eighth-, tenth-, and twelfth-graders from nationally representative samples of schools for the years 1991 through 1999. It comes from the Monitoring the Future project (1999). It is noteworthy that the prevalence of youth smoking went up from 1991 to 1996 at all grades and, despite considerable activity designed to reduce it, adolescent smoking prevalence is still higher than it was in 1993 for 8th and 10th graders and is higher than it was in 1996 for 12th graders.

Table 1. Trends in Prevalence of Cigarettes for Eighth-, Tenth-, and
Twelfth-grade Students

	'91	'92	'93	'94	'95	'96	'97	'98	'99	'98–'99 change
Lifetime										
8th grade	44	45	45	46	46	49	47	46	44	−1.6
10th grade	55	54	56	57	58	61	60	58	58	−0.1
12th grade	63	62	62	62	64	64	65	65	65	−0.7
30-Day										
8th grade	14	16	17	19	19	21	19	19	18	−1.6s
10th grade	21	22	25	25	28	30	30	28	26	−1.9
12th grade	28	28	30	31	34	34	37	35	35	−0.5
Daily										
8th grade	7.2	7	8.3	8.8	9.3	10	9	8.8	8.1	−0.7
10th grade	13	12	14	15	16	18	18	16	16	0.1
12th grade	19	17	19	19	22	22	25	22	23	0.7

Notes: Ns vary from 13,600 to 18,600
Level of significance of difference between the two years indicated = .05
Source: Data adapted from "Trends in Annual and 30-day Prevalence of Use of Various Drugs for 8th,
10th, 12th Graders, 1991–99, The Monitoring the Future Study, 1999.

The Relationship between Smoking and Other
Problem Behaviors

There is an enormous amount of research showing that smoking is correlated with engagement in other problem behaviors including all forms of
substance use, anti-social behavior, and high risk sexual behavior, as well
as academic failure (e.g., Biglan & Smolkowski, in press).

Willard and Schoenborn (1995) present data on the co-occurrence of
cigarette smoking and other behaviors from the 1992 National Health Interview Survey of Youth Risk Behavior (NHIS-YRBS; National Center for
Health Statistics, 1996). The survey is "a continuous, nationwide, household interview survey of the civilian, non-institutionalized population of
the United States" conducted by the National Center for Health Statistics.
The Center interviewed 10,645 persons aged 12 to 21 years.

They reported the proportion of current smokers (one or more
cigarettes in the last month) who engaged in each of a range of problem
behaviors. The behaviors that co-occurred with smoking to a significant
degree are presented in Table 2. Smoking was not significantly related to
cocaine use, due to the unreliability of the reports for Never Smokers. However, 3.5% of current smokers reported cocaine use and only 0.2% of never
smokers did.

Table 2. The Co-occurrence of Smoking and Other Problem Behaviors

Problem behavior	Current smoking (SE)	Never smoker (SE)
Drank alcohol in past month	74.4 (1.11)	23.0 (1.02)
Five or more drinks in row	50.3 (1.22)	9.5 (.69)
Used marijuana in past month	26.5 (1.02)	1.5 (.025)
Smokeless tobacco in past month (boys only)	28.1 (1.76)	4.1 (0.52)
Carried a weapon	25.6 (1.12)	9.5 (0.59)
Physical fight in past year	54.7 (1.09)	29.0 (0.86)
Ever had sexual intercourse	80.0 (0.99)	41.4 (1.40)

Source: Data adapted from "Trends in Annual and 30-day Prevalence of Use of Various Drugs for 8th, 10th, 12th Graders, 1991–99, by The Monitoring the Future Study, 1999.

It is possible that the onset of smoking makes engagement in other problem behaviors more likely; the relationships between smoking and other problems has often been cited as another justification for efforts to prevent adolescent smoking. The evidence on this point is equivocal. Smoking may change adolescents in ways that make them more susceptible to the reinforcement of other substances. It could also be that for the young smoker, the behavior of smoking is associated with rule violation such that initiation of smoking desensitizes the young person to other forms of rule violation. In any case, it is possible that preventing smoking could help to prevent other problem behaviors.

Interventions to Prevent Adolescent Tobacco Use

School-Based Interventions

School-based smoking prevention programs are perhaps the most extensively researched method of reducing adolescent tobacco use. For example, Rooney and Murray's (1996) meta-analysis reviewed 131 studies of the effects of school-based programs and Tobler and colleagues' meta-analysis (Tobler, Roona, Ochshorn, Marshall, Streke, & Stackpole 2000) included 207 studies. The evidence suggests that certain types of school-based programs can have a small but significant effect on adolescent cigarette use. Rooney and Murray (1996) found that the average size of the effect of school-based programs on cigarette smoking was .10 standard deviations. That is, students receiving the program were on average .1 standard deviations lower on measures of smoking than were students not receiving the program.

Tobler and Stratton (1997) conducted a meta-analysis of tobacco prevention studies that distinguished "interactive" and "non-interactive" programs. The non-interactive programs were ones involving little interaction among students and a focus on increasing knowledge and affecting attitudes. The interactive programs included teaching skills for resisting social influences to use tobacco, education about the norms against tobacco use, and opportunities to practice skills and interact with other students while working on these topics. Among interactive programs evaluated in high quality experiments, the average effect size was .29, while for noninteractive programs it was −.06. Thus, the programs that appear most effective are those that have components addressing social influences to smoke, including teaching refusal skills, using peer leaders, and giving students the feedback that fewer young people smoke than adolescents typically believe (Glynn, 1993; Tobler et al., 2000; USDHHS, 1994). There is some evidence that such programs can also prevent smokeless tobacco use (Severson & Biglan, 1989; Severson et al., 1991; Sussman, Dent, Stacy, Hodgson et al., 1993).

After reviewing the evidence on school-based tobacco prevention programs, the Centers for Disease Control and Prevention identified two programs that were especially effective in reducing tobacco use. They are the Life Skills Training program developed by Botvin and colleagues (Botvin, Baker, Dusenbury, Tortu, & Botvin, 1990; Botvin & Dusenbury, 1987; Botvin, Eng, & Williams, 1980; Botvin & Wills, 1992) and Sussman and colleagues' program Towards No Tobacco Use (TNT; Dent et al., 1995; Sussman, Dent, Stacy, Hodgson et al., 1993; Sussman, Dent, Stacy, Sun et al., 1993). The CDC recommends these programs nationwide.

We cannot assume, however, that even well validated programs will be effective when they are widely implemented. First, the effects obtained in carefully controlled studies are modest (Rooney & Murray, 1996) and the effects of such programs will decrease unless researchers carefully manage their implementation (Glasgow, Vogt, & Boles, 1999). A recent review by Tobler et al. (2000) provides empirical evidence in support of this assertion. She found that the larger and more recent studies of school-based programs were less likely to obtain significant effects on smoking. Apparently, as the field has moved to effectiveness trials involving program implementation in many schools (Flay, 1986), replicating the effects of these programs has become more difficult. The implication is that school districts that implemented even well researched programs will need to ensure careful training and high quality implementation of the programs and will need to continue to monitor adolescent tobacco use to be sure that the programs are having their desired effect.

Policies Affecting Tobacco Use

SCHOOL POLICY. Outside of the home, the principal environment of adolescents is the school. The school environment prescribes social norms—either directly or indirectly—through school policies, teacher expectations and behavior, and peer group action. The school has the opportunity to promote tobacco-free norms, counter pro-tobacco messages, and create a health-promoting environment.

School policies can affect tobacco use behavior. Pentz et al. (1989) examined the impact of school smoking policies on more than 4,000 adolescents in 23 schools in California. The schools' written smoking policies were evaluated on whether they banned smoking on school grounds, restricted students leaving school grounds, banned smoking near school, and included an education program on smoking prevention. Schools that had policies in all these areas, and emphasized prevention and cessation, had significantly lower smoking rates than did schools with fewer policies. Similarly, Elder et al. (1996) reported that, in their evaluation of 96 schools in four states, implementation and enforcement of school policies appears to be a crucial part of a school-based intervention, and must be tailored to political and regional factors affecting a specific school district. In sum, schools can create powerful environments for promoting nonsmoking norms, and school policy development is recommended as an integral part of a tobacco prevention program (Glynn, 1993).

Recent national efforts have worked to promote and require "tobacco-free school policies," but few evaluations of these efforts have been conducted. Reports from national surveys (National School Boards Association, 1989) and from schools within Colorado (Colorado State University Cooperative Extension, 1993) and Minnesota (Minnesota Department of Health, 1991) indicate that restrictive smoking policies can gain wide acceptance and support. Drawing on reviews of existing policies and evaluation research, several authors have identified key characteristics of effective smoking control policies for schools (Brink, Simons-Morton, Harvey, Parcel, & Ternan, 1988; DiFranza, 1989; National School Boards Association, 1989; Rashak, Olsen, Speark, & Haggerty, 1986). Most of these have been incorporated into the U.S. Department of Education's Policy Statement 702 (effective March 1998), which established guidelines for tobacco-free schools.

COMMUNITY POLICY.   Changes in tobacco policy at the community level may be expected to have an impact on youth tobacco use within the school cluster neighborhood (Lewit, Hyland, Kerrebrock, & Cummings, 1997). However, little is known about the impact of community policy change. Lewit et al. (1997) found that communities with policies limiting adolescent access to tobacco had lowered rates of tobacco use, but that policies prohibiting smoking in public places or in schools were not associated with a reduction in adolescent tobacco use or intentions to use. Apparently, no one has evaluated the impact of laws prohibiting minors from possessing tobacco, although these laws exist in many states (Jacobson & Wasserman, 1997).

Reducing Illegal Sales of Tobacco to Young People

Widespread efforts to reduce illegal sales of tobacco to young people are underway, due to the clear evidence that easy access to tobacco is a factor that contributes to the onset and continued use of tobacco by adolescents (Forster & Wolfson, 1998). There have now been a sufficient number of studies to allow the identification of more and less effective strategies for reducing illegal tobacco sales. Merchant education, where merchants are simply informed about the law and asked to comply, has been found to produce no large or lasting effects (Altman, Foster, Rasenick-Douss, & Tye, 1989; Altman, Rasenick-Douss, Foster, & Tye, 1991). A program of rewarding clerks for not selling and reminding them of the law if they did sell has been shown to significantly reduce level of sales (Biglan, Henderson et al., 1995; Biglan, Ary, Koehn et al., 1996). Increased enforcement of the law has shown clear results in reducing illegal sales (Forster & Wolfson, 1998; Gemson et al., 1998; Jason, Billows, Schnopp-Wyatt, & King, 1996). Forster and Wolfson (1998) showed that systematic efforts to influence communities to adopt strong anti-sale ordinances could bring about stronger laws and significant reductions in sales.

Unfortunately, the degree to which reducing illegal tobacco sales will reduce adolescent smoking is less clear. The best evidence comes from the study by Forster and Wolfson (1998) in which 14 small Minnesota communities were randomly assigned to a control condition or to an intervention in which a community organizer led a process of pushing for the adoption and enforcement of local ordinances against illegal sales. Illegal sales decreased significantly in both intervention and control communities. Adolescent smoking was significantly lower in intervention communities than in control communities. In a non-experimental study, Jason, Ji, Anes, and Birkhead (1991) found that adolescent smoking prevalence was reduced when sales were curtailed, and several other such studies have reported similar findings (Forster & Wolfson, 1998). However, Rigotti et al. (1997) did not find that adolescent smoking behavior declined even though they produced a substantial reduction in illegal sales in target communities.

Youth Anti-Tobacco Activities

As summarized in the 1994 Surgeon General's Report (USDHHS, 1994), there is voluminous evidence that peers are the most proximal influence on adolescent tobacco use. In essence, the evidence shows that peers who also use tobacco prompt most tobacco use initiation (Friedman, Lichtenstein, & Biglan, 1985). Peers influence adolescent tobacco use in two ways. First, association with peers who smoke makes it more likely that a young person will also smoke. Secondly, there is evidence that adolescents who associate with deviant peers are more likely to smoke even when scientists control for the smoking of those peers (Biglan, Duncan, Ary, & Smolkowski, 1995).

All school-based programs shown to prevent tobacco use include components targeting the influence of peers on tobacco use onset (USDHHS, 1994). Commonly found components aimed at peer influences include: (a) refusal skills training (e.g., Botvin et al., 1980; Botvin & Wills, 1992; Botvin, 1996; Pentz et al., 1989); (b) feedback to young people about the actual proportion of their peers who use tobacco (to counter the common perception that adolescent tobacco use is higher than it really is; Hansen & Evans, 1982; Hansen & Graham, 1991; Hansen & Malotte, 1986; Perry, Kelder, Murray, & Klepp, 1992); (c) public commitments from youth not to use tobacco (Biglan, Duncan et al., 1995; Perry et al., 1992); and (d) using peer leaders to conduct some classroom prevention activities (Perry et al., 1992; Perry & Grant, 1988).

However, there seem to be inherent limits on the degree to which peer influences can be counteracted within a classroom setting. School-based programs miss some high-risk students who tend to be less involved in school than their lower-risk peers. Even those high-risk students who do attend classes regularly can be expected to be more resistant to influence attempts coming either from adults or from higher-status students. Moreover, impact on peer influences is limited by the amount of classroom time that is generally available for prevention programs.

Prevention activities outside the classroom that target peer influences are becoming widespread (e.g., Biglan et al., 2000; Pechmann, 1997) and there is some evidence that involving young people in anti-tobacco activities can influence them to become more negative about tobacco use (Biglan, Ary, Yudelson et al., 1996).

Mobilizing Parental Influences on Adolescent Tobacco Use

Parental influences on adolescent smoking have been extensively studied, primarily by examining the relationship between parental smoking and adolescent smoking. A summary of evidence in the Surgeon General's Report on adolescent tobacco use (USDHHS, 1994) concludes that parents who smoke are more likely to have children who smoke, although this relationship is not strong. However, the possibility that parents might prevent adolescent tobacco use by communicating nonuse expectations and preventing youths' association with deviant peers has received little attention from tobacco control researchers.

A number of studies have shown that parenting practices influence adolescent engagement in the entire range of problem behaviors. They include tobacco, alcohol, and illicit drug use (Ary, Duncan, Duncan, & Hops, 1999; Biglan, Mrazek, Carnine, & Flay, in press; Biglan, Duncan et al., 1995); high-risk sexual behavior (Biglan, Metzler et al., 1990; Biglan, Noell, Ochs, & Smolkowski, 1995; Metzler, Noell, Biglan, & Ary, 1994); and academic failure (Patterson, DeBaryshe, & Ramsey, 1989). The parenting practices that appear to influence youth problem behavior are setting effective limits around problem behaviors and activities that lead to problem behaviors, and promoting alternative pro-social behavior. Parents make it less likely that their children will drift into problem behaviors if they prevent them from associating with peers who engage in these behaviors. They can do this by monitoring their children's associations with deviant peers and making and enforcing rules about where and with whom children spend free time (Ary et al., 1999; Biglan, Mrazek et al., in press; Biglan, Duncan et al., 1995; Biglan, Henderson et al., 1995; Biglan et al., 1990; Biglan & Smolkowski, in press; Duncan, Duncan, Biglan, & Ary, 1998; Irvine, Biglan, Smolkowski, Metzler, & Ary, 1999; Metzler, Noell, & Biglan, 1992; Metzler et al., 1994). Thus, effective limit setting can contribute directly to preventing experimentation with tobacco and other problem behaviors.

Biglan, Ary, Yudelson et al. (1996) found that school-prompted parent-child interactions about tobacco use could influence adolescents' perceptions that their parents do not want them to use tobacco. Middle school students received quizzes about tobacco use to take home to their parents. The activity increased both youth and parental knowledge about the harmful effects of tobacco use and induced more attitudes that are negative toward tobacco use.

Taken together, these findings suggest that parents need to be encouraged to communicate with their children that they do not want them to use tobacco and to set limits on activities that would put their children at risk to experiment with tobacco.

Adolescent Cessation

Few studies have examined adolescent smoking cessation, but researchers agree that a comprehensive program to reduce adolescent tobacco use must include efforts to promote cessation among those who have already initiated tobacco use (Lynch & Bonnie, 1994; Sussman, Lichtman, Ritt, & Pallonen, 1999; USDHHS, 1994). Sussman et al. (1999) propose that, while prevention appears most efficacious among younger, less-frequent tobacco users, cessation appears appropriate for older, heavier users who are further along the stages of change. There is also evidence that adolescents develop nicotine dependency and many adolescents experience withdrawal like that of adult smokers (McNeil, West, Jarvis, Jackson, & Bryant, 1986). Adolescent cessation programs have the advantage of stopping the habitual use of tobacco products before physical consequences accumulate in the rapidly growing and maturing body, and possibly before the habit becomes so ingrained as to make quitting more difficult (USDHHS, 1994).

Unfortunately, there are few published studies of adolescent cessation of either cigarettes or smokeless tobacco, and those that are available vary considerably in quality; many are anecdotal or descriptive accounts of programs. In reviewing 17 studies of adolescent cessation published between 1984 and 1997, Sussman indicates that 10 studies reported successful cessation at follow-up, but with a modest (12%) success rate (Sussman et al., 1999). Other sources of information on adolescent cessation include national probability studies on youth cessation patterns, convenience samples that survey self-initiated cessation, and reports from adolescent prevention programs that determine treatment effects on youth who were smoking or chewing at baseline (Lynch & Bonnie, 1994; USDHHS, 1994).

The Youth Risk Behavior Survey (YRBS) and the High School Seniors Survey (sponsored by the National Institute on Drug Abuse) both report a significant proportion (42%–47%) of high school smokers who want to stop smoking and 39% who have tried to quit at least once (Morbidity and Mortality Weekly Report, 2000). In the 1989 Teenage Attitudes & Practices Survey, 74% of 12- to 18-year-old smokers reported they had thought seriously about quitting, 64% had tried to quit smoking, and 49% had tried to quit in the previous six months (Allen, Moss, Giovino, Shopland, & Pierce, 1993).

Media Campaigns

Pechmann (1997) provides a recent and comprehensive summary of the evidence regarding the value of anti-tobacco advertising in preventing adolescent use. The best available evidence comes from experimental evaluations in which anti-tobacco advertising was compared with a no-media condition. Two of those studies (Flynn et al., 1992; 1994; Perry et al., 1992) showed that anti-tobacco ads, when combined with a school-based program, were associated with significant reductions in adolescent smoking. The third study (Bauman, LaPrelle, Brown, Koch, & Padgett, 1991) did not find an effect. Pechmann (1997) concludes that the Bauman study may not have had an effect because it was advertised less, was restricted to radio ads, and was not combined with a school-based program. She argues that ads need to continue for several years, must present a new portfolio of ads each year to maintain student interest, and must reach youth by the time they are in the sixth grade.

Pechmann (1997) also reviews the evidence from tracking the prevalence of adolescent tobacco use before, during, and after state- or nationwide anti-smoking media campaigns. She notes that, in such quasi-experimental studies, it is difficult to be certain whether changes in the prevalence of smoking are due to the ad campaign. However, she concludes that California ad campaigns have had limited impact on adolescent smoking, possibly because few of the ads targeted adolescents. There was no evidence that a campaign in Minnesota affected adolescent smoking. An ad campaign in Canada was associated with a substantial drop in adolescent smoking (e.g., from 8% among 11- to 13-year-old English-speaking children to just 2%). However, that campaign was accompanied by a substantial increase in the tax on cigarettes, a ban on cigarette advertising, systematic increases in school-based programs, and the availability of youth anti-tobacco activities.

Pechmann (1997) reviews evidence suggesting that the amount of money spent targeting adolescents and the amount of money being spent on tobacco marketing are both factors that influence adolescent tobacco use. Studies of the influence of tobacco marketing indicate that expenditures on tobacco marketing are a potent influence on adolescent smoking (Gilpin & Pierce, 1997; Pierce & Gilpin, 1995).

In sum, research on the effects of anti-tobacco advertising on adolescents remains limited. There is still considerable controversy regarding the types of ads that are effective (Goldman & Glantz, 1998, Pechmann & Ratneshwar, 1994) and even whether anti-tobacco ads can affect the prevalence of adolescent smoking.

There is also a question of whether anti-tobacco ads targeting adults can influence young people not to use tobacco. Pechmann's analysis (1997) makes this seem unlikely. She notes that in states where ads targeted adults but were less aimed toward adolescents, effects were shown for adults but not for adolescents. It is possible, however, that ads specifically attempting to influence adults to discourage adolescent smoking could motivate adults to support prevention efforts (e.g., Goldman & Glantz, 1998).

Tobacco Pricing

The price of tobacco products influences adolescent initiation of smoking. There is evidence that adolescents are more sensitive to price than are adults, at least as far as decisions to continue to smoke are concerned (Farrelly & Bray, 1998; Lewit et al., 1997; Tauras & Chaloupka, 1998). With respect to smoking initiation, Lantz et al. (1999), in a comprehensive review of both longitudinal (Dee & Evans, 1998) and cross-sectional (Douglas & Hariharan, 1994) studies, conclude that there is a significant and negative impact of cigarette taxes upon smoking initiation, after controlling for individual variables predictive of demand. Thus, states and communities should be encouraged to increase the price of tobacco through taxation. In recent years, a number of states have increased their tobacco tax and have dedicated a portion of the revenue to programs to reduce tobacco use.

Project Sixteen: A Randomized Controlled Trial of A Community Intervention to Prevent Adolescent Tobacco Use

We recently completed an experimental evaluation of a comprehensive community-wide program to prevent adolescent tobacco use that incorporates many of the interventions described above (Biglan et al., 2000). We randomly assigned eight pairs of small Oregon communities to receive a school-based prevention program or the school-based program plus the community intervention. The school-based program was Project PATH, which contained the chief components of interactive programs noted above. The curriculum consists of nine levels of instruction. The first four levels were developed for use in grades six through nine. They included materials and videos designed to complement the health education programs in those grade levels. The other levels, developed for the high school curriculum, addressed issues relating to tobacco in health, social studies, biology, and English classes. Specific curriculum components included: (a) health facts and the effect of smoking; (b) refusal skills training for dealing with the social pressures to smoke, chew, use illegal drugs, or engage in antisocial behavior; (c) video-assisted instruction in presenting key concepts and modeling refusal skills; (d) public commitment activities allowing students to clarify their opinions regarding tobacco use; and (e) peer-led discussions and skills practice activities. In a randomized controlled trial, there was evidence that the PATH curriculum, when compared to existing standard health education curricula, reduced the rate of cigarette smoking among adolescents who reported cigarette use before the intervention.

Effects were assessed among seventh and ninth graders through five annual surveys of the prevalence of self-reported smoking and smokeless tobacco use in the month before assessment. The community intervention included four components: (a) media advocacy, (b) youth anti-tobacco activities, (c) family communications about tobacco use, and (d) reducing youth access to tobacco.

The Community Intervention

A paid community coordinator with youth and adult volunteers from the community conducted the community intervention. We defined each component of the intervention by a written module that provides a menu of activities and instructions on how to implement a particular activity. The Advocacy Institute created the Media Advocacy Module for the National Cancer Institute. It provides a set of strategies for publicizing the tobacco problem. An effort was made to influence adults in the community to support efforts to prevent adolescent tobacco use. The effort included newspaper articles and presentations to local civic groups, fact sheets about the problem of adolescent tobacco use that were mailed to community leaders, printed messages on sports programs, paid ads or public service announcements on the radio, billboards at sports fields, and written messages on local cable access "reader boards." The level of these activities in communities was monitored through weekly reports from community coordinators in order to maintain a high rate of communications to as many adults in the community as possible.

The Youth Anti-Tobacco Module provided community coordinators with a menu of activities that would engage young people in anti-tobacco activities. Community coordinators and youth were encouraged to use specified activities, to adapt them to their situation, or to make up entirely new activities. There were eight types of activities: Planning, Creative (e.g., sidewalk art, t-shirt design), Policy Review and Revision, Trade-Ins (tobacco promotion items traded for anti-tobacco items), Giveaways (e.g., t-shirts, posters, stickers, balloons), Games (e.g., a "Knock Down Joe Camel" booth at a health fair), Academic (presentations by community coordinators in classrooms, peer run quizzes), and Other (e.g., participation in parades). An effort was made to recruit young people who seemed particularly at risk to use tobacco.

The Family Communications Module describes activities designed to get parents to communicate to their children that they do not want them to use tobacco. The activities included the distribution to parents of pamphlets about preventing adolescent tobacco use, a student-administered quiz of a parent concerning tobacco use, and letters to parents from prominent community leaders advocating that they complete the tobacco quiz with their child.

The ACCESS Module consists of a five-component program to motivate store clerks not to sell tobacco to minors. The components are: (a) mobilization of community support, (b) merchant education, (c) rewards to clerks for not selling and reminders to those who sell, (d) positive publicity about clerks' refusals to sell, and (e) feedback to store owners or managers about the extent of their sales to adolescents. Reward and reminder visits occurred every two or three weeks until the rates of illegal sales had substantially reduced. Their frequency was then curtailed, though they continued over the duration of the intervention. The program was found to significantly decrease sales in the first four communities in which we intervened (Biglan, Henderson et al., 1995) and those effects were replicated in the other four communities (Biglan, Ary, Koehn et al., 1996).

Given the evidence that research-based programs of this sort often are not effective when widely disseminated, it is important to stress that the program was implemented with careful attention to the quality and quantity of intervention activity in each community. Community coordinators were required to provide weekly reports of their work on each of the youth anti-tobacco, family communications, and access activities. The most frequent activities were youth anti-tobacco activities. Across the three years of intervention activity, the community coordinators reported an average of 10.12, 13.63, and 12.12 youth anti-tobacco activities per month. They reported 3.2, 2.9, and 1.9 youth access activities per month. Finally, 3.9, 1.6, and 0.8 family communications activities were reported each month. We would not expect other communities to achieve the same effects unless they achieved these levels of activity. In addition, they are unlikely to achieve these levels of activity without a system for the ongoing monitoring of implementation.

Effects of the Intervention

The Community Intervention had significant effects on the monthly prevalence of cigarette use at Times 2 and 5 and the effect approached significance at Time 4. The intervention affected the prevalence of smokeless tobacco among ninth grade boys at Time 2, with smokeless use decreasing in Community Intervention communities but not in control communities. There was also a significant effect on the slope of alcohol use among ninth graders. Over the years of the intervention, ninth grade alcohol use increased in control communities but not in intervention communities. Finally, there was evidence that marijuana use was affected by the intervention.

Research on Access Reduction

As part of Project Sixteen, we conducted interrupted time-series experimental evaluations of a positive reinforcement approach to reducing illegal sales of tobacco (Biglan, Ary et al., 1996; Biglan, Henderson et al., 1995). The intervention included rewards for clerks who refused to sell to minors and publicity about clerks who received rewards. It was evaluated in a series of multiple baseline designs in which illegal sales were monitored repeatedly in multiple communities and the intervention was introduced in one community at a time. The intervention produced a sharp reduction in the extent of sales in all but one community. The average proportion of outlets willing to sell dropped from 57% to 22% after the intervention was introduced.

Since Oregon Tobacco Control grants to counties were first awarded in the fall of 1997, we have disseminated our access intervention model to 11 counties. In four of those counties, we contracted with County Public Health Departments to conduct the entire program ourselves. In the remaining seven counties that adopted our model, we conducted training workshops for Public Health staff and/or County Tobacco-Free Coalition members. Level of implementation in each county is measured by (a) degree of community support, (b) percentage of stores in the county that received Reward and Reminder visits, (c) number of Reward and Reminder visits conducted, (d) number of youth and adult volunteers who participated, (e) number and value of rewards donated, and (f) amount of media coverage about the program.

In all four counties where we contracted to undertake the entire intervention, we replicated the results found in our earlier work. In the seven counties where we simply conducted training, we replicated those results in three counties, and two counties have just recently begun the campaign. We believe that variance in results can be attributed to differences in level of commitment of staff time to the effort.

Other Community Interventions

These results suggest that comprehensive community-wide interventions can be of value in preventing adolescent tobacco use and may affect other substance use. They are consistent with evidence from other studies of comprehensive community-wide interventions. Pentz and colleagues (1989) reported the evaluation of a comprehensive community intervention to affect tobacco and other substance use. The program included a school-based program, media directed at parents and children, efforts to mobilize parental influences against substance use, and changes in school and community policies. We found that combining school-based programs with mass media and programs aimed at parents and community leaders can have a greater effect on tobacco and other substance use than providing mass media and parent and community organizing alone.

Perry et al. (1992) compared two communities, one of which received the Minnesota Heart Health program targeting adult cardiovascular health plus a three-year classroom-based prevention program that began when students were in sixth grade. The other community did not receive an intervention. Students in the community receiving the intervention had a significantly lower prevalence of smoking at each year of assessment, through 12th grade.

In the North Karelia Project, an intensive classroom-based smoking prevention program was provided to students in two schools in communities that were also receiving a community-wide comprehensive cardiovascular risk reduction program. Training and materials were provided to the rest of the schools in the county, but project staff did not provide the intervention in these schools. Changes in smoking in the two target schools and two other schools in the county were compared with changes in two schools in a county that received no intervention. Two years after the initiation of the program, the two targeted schools had significantly lower increases in smoking prevalence than did students in the comparison schools.

Although the community trials have varied in the components that they included, they do provide suggestive evidence that greater reductions in adolescent tobacco use can be achieved when community components are added to a school-based intervention. In particular, it would appear that community-wide publicity in support of tobacco reduction may be of value and that involving parents and young people in anti-tobacco activities and reducing adolescents' easy access to tobacco may contribute to reductions in use.

The Potential to Prevent Adolescent Tobacco Use

Existing evidence shows very clearly that it is possible to prevent many adolescents from smoking. Reducing tobacco use among our nation's adolescents will require a concerted and coordinated effort that makes use of everything we have learned. All schools should adopt and implement effective programs approved by the CDC as effective prevention programs and tobacco prevention should be integrated into drug prevention programs aimed at youth. We should continue our efforts to change the social norms and acceptability of tobacco use. Media campaigns can be effective in educating youth and parents about the health risks, promote a tobacco-free environment, and counter the sales promotions of the tobacco industry. Tobacco-free policies should be adopted and enforced to ensure that all public places are smoke-free. Schools need to take a strong position of enforcing rules for a tobacco-free environment, and support to aiding cessation for youth already smoking.

Parents need to be included in the prevention effort and creative ways are needed to help parents set and communicate clear standards for not using tobacco products (even if they are smokers). Other efforts that have proven effective involve a wider context for social action, as we know that increasing the price of tobacco products through taxation can reduce consumption and demand for these products. Reducing access to tobacco can be another deterrent. Access reduction will be facilitated by getting better enforcement of existing laws, publishing names of stores that sell to minors, and passing more stringent laws such as licensing vendors through local ordinances.

During this historic time, knowledge about preventing the use of tobacco can help to significantly reduce the disease and death associated with tobacco use. The master settlement with the tobacco industry (King & Siegel, 2001; Turner-Bowker & Hamilton, 2000), increasing support for legislation to control tobacco sales to minors, proven prevention programs for school adoption, and increases in the tax on tobacco provide an opportunity to implement what is known about the prevention of tobacco in every community.

References

Allen, K., Moss, A.J., Giovino, G.A., Shopland, D.R., & Pierce, J.P. (1993). Teenage tobacco use: Data estimates from the teenage attitudes and practices survey, United States, 1989. *Advance Data, 224,* 1–20.

Altman, D.G., Foster, V., Rasenick-Douss, L., & Tye, J.B. (1989). Reducing the illegal sale of cigarettes to minors. *Journal of the American Medical Association, 261,* 80–83.

Altman, D.G., Rasenick-Douss, L., Foster, V., & Tye, J.B. (1991). Sustained effects of an educational program to reduce sales of cigarettes to minors. *American Journal of Public Health, 81,* 891–893.

Ary, D.V., Duncan, T.E., Duncan, S.C., & Hops, H. (1999). Adolescent problem behavior: The influence of parents and peers. *Behaviour Research and Therapy, 37,* 217–230.

Ary, D.V. Lichtenstein, E., & Severson, H.H. (1987). Smokeless tobacco use among male adolescents: Patterns, correlates, predictors, and the use of other drugs. *Preventive Medicine, 16,* 385–401.

Bauman, K.E., LaPrelle, J., Brown, J.D., Koch, G.G., & Padgett, C.A. (1991). The influence of three mass media campaigns on variables related to adolescent cigarette smoking: Results of a field experiment. *American Journal of Public Health, 81,* 597–604.

Biglan, A., Ary, D.V., Koehn, V., Levings, D., Smith, S., Wright, Z., et al. (1996). Mobilizing positive reinforcement in communities to reduce youth access to tobacco. *American Journal of Community Psychology, 24,* 625–638.

Biglan, A., Ary, D.V., Smolkowski, K., Duncan, T.E., & Black, C. (2000). A randomized controlled trial of a community intervention to prevent adolescent tobacco use. *Tobacco Control, 9,* 24–32.

Biglan, A., Ary, D.V., Yudelson, H., Duncan, T.E., Hood, D., James, L., et al. (1996). Experimental evaluation of a modular approach to mobilizing anti-tobacco influences of peers and parents. *American Journal of Community Psychology, 24,* 311–339.

Biglan, A., Duncan, T.E., Ary, D.V., & Smolkowski, K. (1995). Peer and parental influences on adolescent tobacco use. *Journal of Behavioral Medicine, 18*, 315–330.

Biglan, A., Gallison, C., Ary, D.V., & Thompson, R. (1985). Expired air carbon monoxide and saliva thiocyanate: Relationships to self-reports of marijuana and cigarette smoking. *Addictive Behaviors, 10*, 137–144.

Biglan, A., Henderson, J., Humphreys, D., Yasui, M., Whisman, R., Black, C., et al. (1995). Mobilizing positive reinforcement to reduce youth access to tobacco. *Tobacco Control, 4*, 42–48.

Biglan, A., Metzler, C.W., Wirt, R., Ary, D.V., Ochs, L.M., French, C., et al. (1990). Social and behavioral factors associated with high-risk sexual behavior among adolescents. *Journal of Behavioral Medicine, 13*, 245–261.

Biglan, A., Mrazek, P., Carnine, D.W., & Flay, B.R. (in press). The integration of research and practice in the prevention of youth problem behaviors. *American Psychologist*.

Biglan, A., Noell, J., Ochs, L., & Smolkowski, K. (1995). Does sexual coercion play a role in high-risk sexual behavior of adolescent and young adult women? *Journal of Behavioral Medicine, 18*, 549–568.

Biglan, A., & Smolkowski, K. (2002). Critical influences on the development of adolescent problem behavior. In D.B. Kandel (Ed.), *Stages and pathways of drug involvement: Examining the gateway hypothesis*. Los Angeles: UCLA Youth Enhancement Service.

Botvin, G.J. (1996). Substance abuse prevention through life skills training. In *Preventing childhood disorders, substance abuse, and delinquency* (pp. 215–240). Thousand Oaks, CA: Sage.

Botvin, G.J., Baker, E., Dusenbury, L., Tortu, S., & Botvin, E.M. (1990). Preventing adolescent drug abuse through a multi-modal cognitive-behavioral approach: Results of a 3-year study. *Journal of Consulting and Clinical Psychology, 58*, 437–446.

Botvin, G.J., & Dusenbury, L. (1987). Life skills training: A psychoeducational approach to substance abuse prevention. In C.A. Maher & J.E. Zins (Eds.), *Psychoeducational interventions in the schools: Methods and procedures for enhancing student competence* (pp. 46–65). Elmsford, NY: Pergamon Press.

Botvin, G.J., Eng, A., & Williams, C.L. (1980). Preventing the onset of cigarette smoking through life skills training. *Preventive Medicine, 9*, 135–143.

Botvin, G.J., & Wills, T.A. (1992). *Personal and social skills training: Cognitive-behavioral approaches to substance abuse prevention*. New York: Cornell University Weill Medical College, Health Behavior Research Group.

Brink, S.G., Simons-Morton, D.G., Harvey, C.M., Parcel, G.S., & Ternan, K.M. (1988). Developing comprehensive smoking control programs in schools. *Journal of School Health, 58*, 177–189.

Centers for Disease Control and Prevention. (1989). *Reducing the health consequences of smoking: 25 years of progress* (DHSS Publication No. CDC 89–8411). Washington, DC: U.S. Department of Health and Human Services.

Centers for Disease Control and Prevention. (1990). Cigarette smoking-attributable mortality and years of potential life cost—United States, 1990. *Morbidity and Mortality Weekly Report, 42*, 645–649.

Colorado State University Cooperative Extension. (1993). *Colorado tobacco-free schools and communities: A collaborative community approach*. Fort Collins: Colorado State University.

Dee, T.S., & Evans, W.N. (1998). *A comment on DeCicca, Kenkel, and Mathios*. Atlanta: Georgia Institute of Technology, School of Economics.

Dent, C.W., Sussman, S., Stacy, A.W., Craig, S., Burton, D., & Flay, B.R. (1995). Two-year behavior outcomes of project Towards No Tobacco Use. *Journal of Consulting and Clinical Psychology, 63*, 676–677.

DiFranza, J.R. (1989). School tobacco policy: a medical perspective. *Journal of School Health, 59*, 398–400.

Douglas, S., & Hariharan, G. (1994). The hazards of starting smoking: Estimates from a split population duration model. *Journal of Health Economics, 13*, 213–230.

Duncan, S.C., Duncan, T.E., Biglan, A., & Ary, D.V. (1998). Contributions of the social context to the development of adolescent substance use: A multivariate latent growth modeling approach. *Drug & Alcohol Dependence, 50*, 57–71.

Elder, J.P., Perry, C.L., Stone, E.J., Johnson, C.C., Yang, M., Edmundson, E.W., et al. (1996). Tobacco use measurement, prediction, and intervention in elementary schools in four states: The CATCH Study. *Preventive Medicine, 25*, 486–494.

Farrelly, M.C., & Bray, J.W. (1998). Response to increases in cigarette prices by race/ethnicity, income, and age groups—United States, 1976–1993. *Morbidity and Mortality Weekly Report, 47*, 605–609.

Flay, B.R. (1986). Efficacy and effectiveness trials (and other phases of research) in the development of health promotion programs. *Preventive Medicine, 15*, 451–474.

Flynn, B.S., Worden, J.K., Secker-Walker, R.H., Badger, G.J., Geller, B.M., & Costanza, M.C. (1992). Prevention of cigarette smoking through mass media intervention and school programs. *American Journal of Public Health, 82*, 827–834.

Flynn, B.S., Worden, J.K., Secker-Walker, R.H., Pirie, P.L., Badger, G.J., Carpenter, J.H., et al. (1994). Mass media and school interventions for cigarette smoking prevention: Effects 2 years after completion. *American Journal of Public Health, 84*, 1148–1150.

Forster, J.L., & Wolfson, M. (1998). Youth access to tobacco: Policies and politics. *Annual Review of Public Health, 19*, 203–235.

Friedman, L.S., Lichtenstein, E., & Biglan, A. (1985). Smoking onset among teens: An empirical analysis of initial situations. *Addictive Behaviors, 10*, 1–13.

Gemson, D.H., Moats, H.I., Watkins, B.X., Ganz, M.I., Robinson, S., & Healton E. (1998). Laying down the law: Reducing illegal tobacco sales to minors in central Harlem. *American Journal of Public Health, 88*, 936–939.

Gilpin, E.A., & Pierce, J.P. (1997). Trends in adolescent smoking initiation in the United States: Is tobacco marketing an influence? *Tobacco Control, 6*, 122–127.

Glasgow, R.E., Vogt, T.M., & Boles, S.M. (1999). Evaluating the public health impact of health promotion interventions: The RE-AIM Framework. *American Journal of Public Health, 89*, 1322-27.

Glynn, T.J. (1993). Improving the health of U.S. children: The need for early interventions in tobacco use. *Preventive Medicine, 22*, 513–19.

Goldman, L.K., & Glantz, S.A. (1998). Evaluation of anti-smoking advertising campaigns. *Journal of American Medical Association, 279*, 772–777.

Hansen, W.B., & Evans, R.I. (1982). Feedback versus information concerning carbon monoxide as an early intervention strategy in adolescent smoking. *Adolescence, 17*, 90–98.

Hansen, W.B., & Graham, J.W. (1991). Preventing alcohol, marijuana, and cigarette use among adolescents: Peer pressure resistance training versus establishing conservative norms. *Preventive Medicine, 20*, 414–430.

Hansen, W.B., & Malotte, C.K. (1986). Perceived personal immunity: The development of beliefs about susceptibility to the consequences of smoking. *Preventive Medicine, 15*, 363–372.

Irvine, A.B., Biglan, A., Smolkowski, K., Metzler, C.W., & Ary, D.V. (1999). The effectiveness of a parenting skills program for parents of middle school students in small communities. *Journal of Consulting and Clinical Psychology, 67*, 811–825.

Jacobson, P.D., & Wasserman, J. (1997). *Tobacco control laws. Implementation and enforcement.* Santa Monica, CA: Rand.

Jason, L.A., Billows, W.D., Schnopp-Wyatt, D.L., & King, C.P. (1996). Reducing illegal sales of cigarettes to minors. *Journal of Applied Behavior Analysis, 29*, 333–344.

Jason, L.A., Ji, P.Y., Anes, M.D., & Birkhead, S.H. (1991). Active enforcement of cigarette control laws in the prevention of cigarette sales to minors. *Journal of the American Medical Association, 266*, 3159–3161.

King, C.I., & Siegel, M. (2001). The master settlement agreement with the tobacco industry and cigarette advertising in magazines. *New England Journal of Medicine, 345*, 504–511.

Lantz, P.M., Jacobson, P.D., Warner, K.D., Wasserman, J., Pollack, H., Berson, J., & Ahlstrom, A. (1999). Investing in youth tobacco control: A review of smoking prevention and control strategies. Unpublished.

Lewit, E.M., Hyland, A., Kerrebrock, N., & Cummings, K.M. (1997). Price, public policy, and smoking in young people. *Tobacco Control, 6*(Suppl. 2), S17–S24.

Lightwood, J.M., Phibbs, C.S., & Glantz, S. (1999). Short-term health and economic benefits of smoking cessation: Low birth weight. *Pediatrics, 104*, 1312–1320.

Lowe, J.B., Balanda, K.P., & Clare, G. (1998). Evaluation of antenatal smoking cessation programs for pregnant women. *Australian and New Zealand Journal of Public Health, 22*, 55–59.

Lynch, B.S., & Bonnie, R.J. (1994). *Growing up tobacco free: Preventing nicotine addiction in children and youths*. Washington, DC: National Academy Press.

McNeil, A.D., West, R.J., Jarvis, M., Jackson, P., & Bryant, A. (1986). Cigarette withdrawal symptoms in adolescent smokers. *Psychopharmacology, 90*, 533–536.

Metzler, C.W., Noell, J., & Biglan, A. (1992). The validation of a construct of high-risk sexual behavior in heterosexual adolescents. *Journal of Adolescent Research, 7*, 233–249.

Metzler, C.W., Noell, J., Biglan, A., & Ary, D. (1994). The social context for risky sexual behavior among adolescents. *Journal of Behavioral Medicine, 17*, 419–438.

Minnesota Department of Health. (1991). *The Minnesota tobacco-use prevention initiative 1989–1990: A report to the 1991 Legislature*. Minneapolis: MN Department of Health.

Monitoring the Future. (1999). Trends in annual and 30-day prevalence of use of various drugs for 8th, 10th, 12th Graders, 1991–99. Retrieved March 28, 2001, from http://monitoringthefuture.org/data/99data.html

Morbidity and Mortality Weekly Report. (2000). Youth Tobacco Surveillance—United States, 1998–1999. *MMWR, 49(SS10)*, 1–93.

Murray, D.M., O'Connell, C.M., Schmid, L.A., & Perry, C.L. (1987). The validity of smoking self-reports by adolescents: A reexamination of the bogus pipeline procedure. *Addictive Behaviors, 12*, 7–15.

Murray, D.M., & Perry, C.L. (1987). The measurement of substance use among adolescents: When is the "bogus pipeline" method needed? *Addictive Behaviors, 12*, 225–233.

National Center for Health Statistics (1996). *Health, United States, 1995*. Hyattsville, MD: Public Health Service.

National School Boards Association. (1989). *Smoke-free schools: A progress report*. Alexandria, VA: National School Boards Association.

Patterson, G.R., DeBaryshe, B.D., & Ramsey, E. (1989). A developmental perspective on antisocial behavior [Special issue]. *American Psychologist, 44*, 329–335.

Pechacek, T.F., Murray, D.M., Luepker, R.V., Mittelmark, M.B., Johnson, C.A., & Shultz, J.A. (1984). Measurement of adolescents smoking behavior: Rationale and methods. *Journal of Behavioral Medicine, 7*, 123–140.

Pechmann, C. (1997). Does anti–smoking advertising combat underage smoking? A review of past practices and research. In M.E. Goldberg, M. Fishbein, & S.E. Middlestadt (Eds.), *Social marketing: Theoretical and practical perspectives* (pp. 189–216). Mahwah, NJ: Lawrence Erlbaum.

Pechmann, C., & Ratneshwar, S. (1994). The effects of anti-smoking and cigarette advertising on young adolescents' perceptions of peers who smoke. *Journal of Consumer Research, 21,* 236–251.

Pentz, M.A., MacKinnon, D.P., Flay, B.R., Hansen, W.B., Johnson, C.A., & Dwyer, J.H. (1989). Primary prevention of chronic diseases in adolescence: Effects of the Midwestern Prevention Project on tobacco use. *American Journal of Epidemiology, 130,* 713–724.

Perry, C.L., & Grant, M. (1988). Comparing peer-led to teacher-led youth alcohol education in four countries. *Alcohol Health and Research World, 12,* 322–336.

Perry, C.L., Kelder, S.H., Murray, D.M., & Klepp, K.I. (1992). Community-wide smoking prevention: Long-term outcomes of the Minnesota Hearth Health Program and the Class of 1989 study. *American Journal of Public Health, 82,* 1210–1216.

Pierce, J.P., & Gilpin, E.A. (1995). A historical analysis of tobacco marketing and the uptake of smoking by youth in the United States: 1890–1977. *Health Psychology, 14,* 500–508.

Rashak, N.E., Olsen, L.K., Speark, A.K., & Haggerty, J.M. (1986). Smoking policies of secondary schools in Arizona. *Journal of School Health, 56,* 180–183.

Rigotti, N.A., DiFranza, J.R., Chang, Y., Tisdale, T., Kemp, B., & Singer, E. (1997). The effect of enforcing tobacco-sales laws on adolescents' access to tobacco and smoking behavior. *The New England Journal of Medicine, 337,* 1044–1051.

Rooney, B.L., & Murray, D.M. (1996). A meta-analysis of smoking prevention programs after adjustment for errors in the unit of analysis. *Health Education Quarterly, 23,* 48–64.

Severson, H.H. & Biglan, A. (1989). Rationale for the use of passive consent in smoking prevention research: Politics, policy, and pragmatics. *Preventive Medicine, 18,* 267–279.

Severson, H.H., Eakin, E.G., Lichtenstein, E., & Stevens, V.J. (1990). The inside scoop on the stuff called snuff: An interview study of 94 adult male smokeless tobacco users. *Journal of Substance Abuse, 2,* 77–85.

Severson, H.H., Glasgow, R., Wirt, R., Zoref, L., Black, C., Biglan, A., et al. (1991). Preventing the use of smokeless tobacco and cigarettes by teens: Results of a classroom intervention. *Health Education Research, 6,* 109–120.

Severson, H.H., Lichtenstein, E., & Gallison, C. (1985). A pinch or a pouch instead of a puff? Implications of chewing tobacco for addictive process. *Bull Psychologists Addictive Behaviors, 4,* 85–92.

Smoking-related deaths and financial costs: Office of technology assessment estimates for 1990. Hearing before the Senate Special Committee on Aging on Preventive health: An ounce of prevention saves a pound of cure, 103rd Cong., 2 (1993) (testimony of R. Herdman, M. Hewitt, & M. Laschober).

Sussman, S., Dent, C.W., Stacy, A.W., Hodgson, C.S., Burton, D., & Flay, B.R. (1993). Project Towards No Tobacco Use: Implementation, process, and post-test knowledge evaluation. *Health Education, 8,* 109–123.

Sussman, S., Dent, C.W., Stacy, A.W., Sun, P., Craig, S., Simon, T.R., et al. (1993). Project Towards No Tobacco Use: 1-Year behavior outcomes. *American Journal of Public Health, 83,* 1245–1250.

Sussman, S., Lichtman, K., Ritt, A., & Pallonen, U. (1999). Effects of thirty-four adolescent tobacco use cessation and prevention trials on regular users of tobacco products. *Substance Use & Misuse 34,* 1469–1505.

Tauras, J.A., & Chaloupka, F.J. (1998). *Price, clean indoor air laws, and cigarette smoking: Evidence from longitudinal data for young adults.* Ann Arbor: University of Michigan.

Tobler, N.S., Roona, M.R., Ochshorn, P., Marshall, D.G., Streke, A.V., & Stackpole, K.M. (2000). School-based adolescent drug prevention programs: 1998 meta-analysis. *Journal of Primary Prevention, 20*(4), 275–336.

Tobler, N.S., & Stratton, H.H. (1997). Effectiveness of school-based drug prevention programs: A meta-analysis of the research. *Journal of Primary Prevention, 18,* 71–128.

Turner-Bowker, D. & Hamilton, W. (2000). *Cigarette advertising expenditures before and after master settlement agreement: Preliminary findings*. Boston: Massachusetts Department of Public Health.

U.S. Department of Health & Human Services. (1989). *Reducing the health consequences of smoking 25 years of progress: a report of the Surgeon General*. Washington, DC: U.S. Department of Health & Human Services.

U.S. Department of Health & Human Services. (1994). *Preventing tobacco use among young people: A report of the Surgeon General*. Washington, DC: Author.

Willard, J.C., & Schoenborn, C.A. (1995). Relationship between cigarette smoking and other unhealthy behaviors among our nation's youth: United States, 1992. *Advance data from vital and health statistics, No. 263*. Hyattsville, MD: National Center for Health Statistics.

Chapter 4

The Prevention of Drug Abuse

Anthony Biglan, Brian Flay, and Sharon L. Foster

This chapter reviews the evidence about preventing the abuse of illicit drugs. During the last 25 years, an enormous amount has been learned about the factors that influence the development of drug-using behavior and the things that can be done to prevent drug use. Sufficient knowledge exists to justify the implementation of prevention programs in schools and communities because school and community-based programs have been shown to prevent drug use and the development of numerous problems that are associated with drug abuse. At the same time, most studies have focused on drug use rather than drug abuse. A new generation of research studies will be needed to determine whether comprehensive prevention programs actually prevent serious forms of substance abuse.

The Problem of Drug Abuse

According to the 1994 National Household Survey on Drug Abuse, an estimated 12.6 million adults had used an illicit drug in the past month (Substance Abuse and Mental Health Services Administration, 1995), with marijuana being the most commonly used drug. Further evidence suggests that this household survey underestimated drug use, because data were collected using interviews (Glantz, Weinberg, Miner, & Colliver, 1999). The 1996 Institute of Medicine (IOM) report cites a study indicating that there were 2.1 million cocaine users and 440,000 to 600,000 heroin users (Rhodes et al. 1995, as cited by IOM, 1996).

Data on adolescent use of illicit drugs come from the Monitoring the Future study (Monitoring the Future, 1999, Table 1b), which has obtained questionnaire reports on drug use from 8th, 10th, and 12th graders for 1991 through 1999. In 1999, 25.9% of 12th graders, 22.1% of 10th graders, and 12.2% of 8th graders reported using at least one illicit drug in the past month. These figures reflect an increasing trend in the use of illicit drugs over the decade of the 90's, particularly marijuana. Another noteworthy aspect of these data is the fact that—in contrast to other drugs—the use of inhalants is greater among eighth graders than among older students. Thus, strategies to prevent inhalant use may need to differ from those to prevent other drug use and abuse.

Teens use other illicit drugs much less often than they use marijuana. Among 12th graders in 1999, 2.6% reported using cocaine, 0.5% heroin, 4.5% amphetamines, and 3.5% hallucinogens. Because school-based surveys do not provide in-depth information about the patterns of drug use, it is unclear what proportion of these users experience serious problems of abuse and dependence. In addition, school-based surveys may underestimate teens' use because serious users may have dropped out of school. Finally, because schools vary widely in numbers of drug users, we can assume that in some schools there are substantially larger numbers of users.

The Distinction between Drug Use and Abuse

Survey research on adolescent drug use typically does not provide sufficient detail about the use of illicit drugs to identify respondents who have abuse or dependence problems. Diagnostic criteria for "Drug Abuse" involve recurrent or continued use of a substance in the face of problems with role fulfillment, interpersonal relations, the law, or physical hazards. For example, according to the DSM-IV (American Psychiatric Association, 1994), the standard for psychiatric diagnosis in the United States, the criteria for the more severe label of "dependence" involve significant impairment in the form of problems in three or more areas. These areas are: tolerance; withdrawal symptoms; compulsive use; difficulty curtailing use; extensive time spent using or coping with the results of using; reduction in social, occupational, or recreational activities due to drug use; and continued use despite evidence that use contributes to physical or psychological illness. However, survey research typically obtains data only about the frequency of use.

This creates two problems for drug abuse research. First, it is unclear to what extent the factors that predict drug *use* also predict the development of drug *abuse* (Glantz et al., 1999). Second, studies of the prevention of adolescent drug use are unable to determine whether interventions prevent abuse. That is, even when a prevention program significantly lowers the prevalence of drug use, one cannot be sure that this translates into the prevention of abuse. For example, the program may deter young people from trying illicit drugs who would not transition to abusive use, but have little impact on multi-problem youths who, as shown below, are most likely to have problems with drug abuse and dependence. We will argue that prevention programs must begin to focus on reducing drug abuse as well as drug use because: (a) we cannot be sure that prevention of drug use also prevents abuse, and (b) drug abuse has serious negative personal, social, and economic consequences.

The Consequences of Drug Abuse

Drug abuse accounts for numerous problems of physical health, psychological well-being, and crime. The 1996 IOM report summarizes the evidence. Among the health consequences associated with drug abuse are HIV/AIDS infections that result from drug users sharing needles, unsafe sexual contacts with infected drug users, and mother to infant transmission of the virus. Injecting drug use may be the number-one risk factor for HIV infection (IOM, 1996). In addition, injection drug users have higher rates of viral and bacterial infections, including hepatitis and pneumonia. Numerous psychiatric disorders are known to co-occur with drug abuse and it is likely that some of them result from or are heightened by drug abuse. Fetal development is impaired by maternal drug use, and children are more likely to be neglected or abused in homes with drug-abusing parents.

Crime and violence have been linked to drug abuse. Some crime results from drug abusers stealing to support drug habits and some stems from the violent nature of the drug distribution system. Acute intoxication with certain drugs may increase the likelihood of violent behavior, although the clearest findings are for alcohol use, which this chapter does not address. The IOM (1996) report reviews evidence that, when drug abuse co-occurs with certain psychiatric disorders, the likelihood of violence rises substantially, especially for lower socioeconomic status males.

Drug use is associated with lower school performance, school dropout, and adolescent delinquency. Among workers, it is associated with greater absenteeism, job turnover, and on-the-job accidents. The degree to which drug abuse actually causes these outcomes is unclear. At a minimum, however, we can safely say that drug abuse in conjunction with other behavioral and psychological difficulties makes certain life problems more likely.

Drug abuse is also economically costly to society. Rice, Kelman, Miller, and Dunmeyer (1990) examined the cost of drug abuse in 1990 dollars. They estimated that the abuse of illicit drugs cost the United States $66 billion per year. It was estimated that $14 billion per year was spent on the direct care of drug abusers. The cost of lost wages due to morbidity and mortality was estimated at $11 billion. Costs due to drug-related crime were estimated at $45.9 billion per year. Finally, the cost due to drug-related AIDS cases for 1990 was estimated at about $6.3 billion per year.

Taking a somewhat different tack, Cohen (1998) estimated the cost over a lifetime of an individual young person who becomes a drug abuser. The costs he considered included resources that are devoted to the drug market that would be spent on other productive activities, the cost of drug treatment, reductions in productivity of drug abusers, medical care, premature death, criminal justice costs, and the cost of additional crime that is due to drug use. Discounting future costs, he concluded that the average lifetime cost of a single young person who becomes a drug abuser is between $370,000 and $970,000. Regardless of whether one considers economic or less easily quantifiable outcomes, drug abuse clearly is a difficulty worth preventing.

The Development of Drug Abuse

Because most etiological studies obtain measures of drug use, not abuse or dependence (Glantz et al., 1999; IOM, 1996), considerably more is known about the factors associated with the development of drug use than the factors associated with the development of drug abuse or dependence. Obviously, a person must use a substance before he or she can become addicted to it. However, factors that influence the development of drug abuse may play little or no role in the initiation of use. In this section, we briefly summarize what is known about behavioral, psychological, and social influences involved in the development of drug use and abuse.

Behavioral and Psychological Factors Related to Drug Use and Abuse

The IOM report (1996) summarizes a wealth of information about behavioral and psychological correlates of drug use. Drug use is most likely among adolescents who are low in academic achievement, more tolerant toward deviance, more rebellious, and less religious. Moreover, it is well established that teens frequently begin use of illicit drugs following the use of tobacco and alcohol (e.g., Kandel, Yamaguchi, & Chen, 1992).

Studies of the relationships between behavioral and psychological variables and drug use pinpoint useful markers of proneness to use drugs. However, they leave open the question of how the young person developed the behavior or psychological factors that precede illicit drug use.

If our goal is to prevent drug use or abuse, we must identify *environments* that could prevent problems such as academic failure and rebelliousness and must evaluate whether doing so does, in fact, lead to less drug use.

Substantial evidence suggests that drug abuse and dependence co-occur with other diagnosable psychological disorders including conduct and oppositional/defiant disorders, anxiety disorders, and depression (Glantz et al., 1999; IOM, 1996). There is, in particular, evidence that drug abuse is very likely among persons with conduct disorder, oppositional defiant disorder, and anti-social personality disorder (Glantz et al., 1999). In general, these diagnoses characterize individuals who are aggressive, disruptive, argumentative, noncompliant with authority, and unconcerned with others' well being. Robins and McEvoy (1990) found that adults who reported any history of drug use were significantly more likely to have drug abuse problems if they had engaged in any one of nine conduct problems (e.g., stealing, skipping school, fighting) as a youth. Most importantly, 80% of the people who reported problems with the use of three or four substances had at least two conduct problems. Conduct problems predicted earlier use of substances, which, in turn, was associated with a greater likelihood of drug abuse. Thus, a large percentage of drug abusers also show significant evidence of conduct problems. This is important because it implies that success in preventing conduct problems could also reduce the number of drug abuse cases.

Peer and Parental Influences on Drug Use

A great deal of research has examined social influences that lead to the development of drug use. The most immediate factor related to drug use is the peer group: many studies have found that association with deviant peers makes it more likely that adolescents will use drugs in the future (e.g., Biglan & Smolkowski, 2002).

This is due partly to adolescents selecting friends who are like them in substance use (Bauman & Ennett, 1996), and partly to how teens influence one another when they interact together. Dishion and colleagues (Dishion, Capaldi, Spracklen, & Li, 1995; Dishion, Eddy, Haas, & Li, 1997; Dishion, Spracklen, Andrews, & Patterson, 1996) directly observed 13- and 14-year-old boys who were at high risk for anti-social behavior while they interacted with a friend. They found that conversations between delinquent boys and their friends were significantly more likely than the conversations of non-delinquent friends to involve sequences in which one boy talked about deviant behavior and the other responded positively. They then found that this "deviancy training" predicted increased substance use, self-reported delinquency, and police-reported violent delinquency two years later. This research provides some direct evidence that adolescent peer interactions reinforce deviant behavior.

Parenting practices also influence the development of drug use. For example, Ary and colleagues (Ary et al., 1999; Ary, Duncan, Duncan, & Hops, 1999) found that high levels of parent-child conflict and low levels of positive parent-child involvement characterized families in which the parents monitored the child's whereabouts infrequently. These low rates of parental monitoring in turn were associated with teens' involvement with deviant peers and various teen problem behaviors, including substance use. These relationships have been replicated with large samples of European American, Mexican American, and Native American male and female adolescents (Barrera, Biglan, Ary, & Li, 2001).

Most studies of peer and parental influences merely link these variables to initial (first-time) drug use or to increases in teens' use of tobacco, alcohol, or other drugs. They do not indicate the extent to which peer and parental factors contribute to the development of drug *abuse* or *dependence*. These factors may play a greater role in the initial use of drugs than in the development of abuse. For example, peers may invite or encourage their friends to use drugs in the context of their social relationships, but whether abuse or dependence develops may also be a function of other risk factors such as biological predispositions to dependence (Glantz et al., 1999; IOM, 1996).

Work at the Oregon Social Learning Center has produced a useful model of the development of anti-social behavior and drug use that appears quite relevant to understanding the development of drug abuse and dependence. Recall that Robins and McEvoy (1990) found that as many as 80% of drug abusers had a history of two or more conduct problems. Patterson, Forgatch, Yoerger, and Stoolmiller (1998) found that such conduct problems are highly predictable from a history of early aggressive behavior. Indeed, 88% of boys who were arrested before age 14 had elevated levels of anti-social behavior at age 9 and 46% of those with high rates of anti-social behavior were arrested prior to age 14. These findings suggest that understanding the developmental pathways involved in the development from early anti-social behavior to early conduct problems would contribute to understanding the development of drug abuse for a large proportion of the drug abusing population.

According to the Oregon Social Learning Center model (Dishion, Capaldi et al., 1995; Patterson, 1999; Patterson, Reid, & Dishion, 1992; Patterson & Yoerger, 1999), aggressive and disruptive behavior in young children occurs in the context of harsh and inconsistent discipline by parents. Much of this work is based on meticulous direct observation of day-to-day parent-child interactions in families' homes. These observations reveal that parents of aggressive boys respond to their son's irritable, aggressive, or noncompliant behavior inconsistently—sometimes by ignoring it, but often by criticizing, ridiculing, commanding, yelling, or hitting (Patterson et al., 1992). Importantly, however, the child's negative behavior often gets the parent to desist—to back down on a command or to stop yelling. Similarly, the parent's behavior occasionally also results in a transient decrease in the child's negative behavior. Thus, an irritable, whiny three-year-old can teach a parent to make few demands of the child simply by whining when asked to do something and ceasing to whine when the parent backs off. Parent and child together train each other to become progressively more negative because these tactics work to stop the other's unpleasant behavior, at least temporarily. The paradox is that, over time, and because of the coercive ways learned to manage others' behavior, negativity in the family escalates rather than declines.

When aggressive boys enter school, their well-developed aggressive repertoires lead to social rejection by non-aggressive peers and their noncompliance in the classroom contributes to academic failure (Patterson, DeBaryshe, & Ramsey, 1989). Furthermore, children who are highly aggressive and uncooperative in school settings are very unlikely to desist from or grow out of such behavior in the absence of a well-organized intervention (Walker, Colvin, & Ramsey, 1995). By late childhood, these young people begin to form friendships with other rejected children. Their parents are not likely to step in and prevent these deviant peer associations because—due to a long history of conflict—parents are loathe to monitor their child's activities or to attempt to set limits on them. Patterson et al. (1989) argue that such deviant peer groups provide a fertile training ground for initiating problem behaviors including substance use and delinquency. Additionally, as noted above, delinquent peers reinforce each other's talk about deviant behavior, propelling the child toward further substance use and delinquency (Dishion, Capaldi et al., 1995; Patterson, Dishion, & Yoerger, 2000).

This analysis clarifies why aggression and conduct disorder are related to drug abuse. Conduct-disordered children are likely to use drugs in the context of their deviant peer group. They are more likely to transition to abuse and dependence because they have few alternative sources of reinforcement (Patterson et al., 1989) and perhaps because the stressful environments in which they live make them more susceptible to the reinforcement of drugs of abuse (Goeders, 1998). Adults who are later diagnosed with anti-social personality disorder are simply aggressive children grown older. They often picked up their drug abusing habits in adolescence (Robins & McEvoy, 1990).

School-Based Curricula to Prevent Drug Abuse

The most commonly employed strategy for preventing drug abuse involves school-based curricula. Numerous curricular interventions have been developed and experimentally evaluated in the last 20 years. All are designed to prevent adolescent use of tobacco, alcohol, and illicit drugs. Much of the impetus for this line of work came from efforts to prevent adolescent tobacco use (e.g., Biglan, Glasgow, Ary, & Thompson, 1987; Biglan, Severson, Ary, & Faller, 1987).

Initial curricula consisted of information about drugs and their effects. Subsequent programs focused on sensitizing young people to the social influences to use substances and providing them with skills for resisting those influences.

A study by Donaldson, Graham, Piccinin, and Hansen (1995) provides a good example of programs that have been developed and helps pinpoint their key ingredients. They compared the effects of giving feedback about norms for substance use among young people with training in skills for resisting peer influences to use substances. They hypothesized that changing norms and providing skills for resisting influences would be an effective combination, but that teaching skills for resisting peer pressures to use drugs without also providing information about the norms against using drugs, might inadvertently give young people the sense that most young people favored using drugs. They randomly assigned public and parochial schools to one of four conditions: (a) information about drugs, (b) information plus resistance skills training, (c) information plus normative education, and (d) information plus resistance skills training and normative education. Information consisted of four 45-minute lessons about health and social consequences of using alcohol and other drugs. Resistance training consisted of four lessons that included a description of likely social pressures, modeling and practicing techniques for resisting those pressures, and parent-child interviews about peer and media pressures to use drugs. Normative education included four lessons about the consequences of drug use and five lessons designed to correct erroneous beliefs about the prevalence and acceptability of drug and alcohol use. A set of additional activities helped students see that fewer students favored use than was generally believed and to make explicit young people's opposition to drug use at that age.

Donaldson et al. (1995) found that in public schools, students who received only resistance skill training had higher estimates of likelihood of offers of drugs after the program than did students in schools receiving the other programs. Students in schools receiving normative education and resistance skills training, however, believed there would be fewer offers than those in other conditions did. In parochial schools, normative education produced lower estimates of the number of offers of drugs and alcohol than did other conditions, but resistance training did not raise those expectations. Additional analyses indicated that students who were more skilled in refusing drugs and alcohol used less alcohol, but only among students who believed that it was not acceptable to drink. However, among students who believed it was acceptable to drink, refusal skills were unrelated to alcohol use. Thus, changing norms, beliefs about the acceptability of substance use, and providing skills for dealing with social influences to use are important in preventing drug use.

Botvin developed a curricular intervention to prevent substance use that has been extensively evaluated and has typically been found to have a significant preventive effect. The program (Life Skills Training) consists of twenty sessions usually delivered in 7th grade with booster sessions delivered in 8th grade. The curriculum covers the consequences of substance use (tobacco, alcohol, and other drugs), the acceptability of use, decision making about use, resistance skill training, self-directed behavior change, techniques for coping with anxiety, communications skills, and general interpersonal and assertiveness skills (Botvin, Baker, Filazzola, & Botvin, 1990). Booster sessions essentially review these themes and provide additional practice of skills.

Botvin (2000) recently reported on a $6^{1}/_{2}$-year follow-up of the effects of Life Skills Training on illicit drug use for a subsample of young people who participated in a study of the program. The study was important because it is one of the few that provides evidence about the effects of such programs on the use of illicit drugs other than marijuana. Botvin (2000) found that those who participated in the program were significantly less likely to use heroin, other narcotics, or hallucinogens than students randomly assigned to control conditions; participants also had lower total reported use of illicit drugs, both when marijuana was included in the total and when it was not. They did not find, however, that the program affected cocaine use. The results provide the strongest evidence to date that curricular-based prevention programs could prevent the use of illicit drugs. Although the data do not document the prevention of the *abuse* of illicit drugs, they come closer to doing so than do other studies, because they show that the program had an impact on the use of drugs that are highly likely to be abused or to meet the criteria for dependence.

The Life Skills program has also been found to have beneficial effects among African American and Hispanic students in an inner city. Botvin, Epstein, Baker, Diaz, and Ifill-Williams (1997) found that at a three-month follow-up, the program had a significant impact on self-reported cigarette, alcohol, and marijuana use and that the level and current use of any drugs was reduced. Thus, it appears that the benefits of the Life Skills programs are not restricted to European American middle class youth.

Meta-analyses of the Effects of Curricular Interventions

Meta-analyses consist of statistical analyses of all of the evaluations of a particular type of intervention. They provide an estimate across studies of the average effect of that intervention. One set of meta-analyses, for example, examined the results of evaluations of the Drug Abuse Resistance Education (DARE) program, probably the most widely disseminated prevention program. These meta-analyses of evaluations of the DARE program indicate that it does not prevent drug use (Ennett, Tobler, Ringwalt, & Flewelling, 1994).

Tobler et al. (2000) provide the most recent meta-analysis of the effects of curricular prevention programs on drug use. For the purposes of their analysis, they divided programs into non-interactive and interactive. Non-interactive programs are ones that rely on lectures and allow little student interaction; they tend to emphasize informational and affective approaches. Interactive programs have a high degree of student activity and interaction, including, for example, the use of peer leaders to conduct lessons and the use of behavior rehearsal to practice skills. Tobler et al. (2000) found that non-interactive programs did not have an effect on self-reported drug use. Studies of interactive programs did have a significant impact on drug use, but those effects were smaller for the larger scale implementations than for the smaller scale studies. This finding points to the possible difficulty of achieving the benefits of these programs when they are widely implemented.

In a similar meta-analysis, Tobler, Lessard, Marshall, Ochshorn, and Roona (1999) evaluated the effects of 37 curricular prevention programs on marijuana use. Non-interactive, lecture-type programs had minimal effects. The interactive programs produced, on average, significant reductions in self-reported marijuana use.

The Value of Curricular Interventions

Our reading of the evidence leads us to the conclusions outlined here. First, curricular interventions that actively involve young people in normative education and social skills training can be of significant benefit in preventing the use of tobacco, alcohol, and marijuana, if they are implemented consistently and well. Second, evidence indicates that positive effects can be achieved among diverse ethnic groups. Third, since the use of licit and illicit drugs precedes the development of drug abuse, it is plausible that these programs can contribute to preventing the *abuse* of illicit drugs. However, further research on this point is needed. Fourth, it is appropriate for schools to implement curricular interventions that have been shown in multiple studies to produce beneficial effects on drug use with students from diverse ethnic and racial groups. The best-supported program appears to be the Life Skills program.

At the same time, evidence that it is difficult to achieve effects with these interventions in large-scale implementations leads us to two additional conclusions. First, ongoing evaluation of substance use among students should be a fundamental feature of a school's efforts to prevent drug use. We cannot assume that even the most well-validated prevention programs will continue to be effective when they come into routine use. Ongoing monitoring of student behavior must be conducted to assess program effects over time. Second, given the relatively modest effects of even the best curricular programs and the many risk factors for drug abuse that are not addressed by curricular interventions, schools and communities must implement additional practices to prevent the development of drug abuse. In the next section, we describe additional practices that may be of benefit.

Beyond Classroom Interventions

Given the many factors that contribute to the development of drug use and abuse, it would be surprising if classroom-based interventions were a sufficient deterrent to drug abuse. Classroom programs can have little effect in altering family influences on drug use. They do not take advantage of media influences on young people. Moreover, for the young people most at risk, they may have limited impact on peer influences. Recall that young people at greatest risk for drug abuse are those who are high in anti-social behavior and have been rejected by non-deviant peers. These young people may be less influenced than others are by information about the normative beliefs of non-deviant peers. Indeed, they are less likely even to be in class when curricular activities occur.

A variety of additional strategies has been considered in trying to prevent drug abuse. They include mass media campaigns, interventions designed to deter drug use by influencing parenting practices, comprehensive community interventions targeting the entire population of adolescents, and interventions targeted at young people at high risk for drug abuse due to high levels of aggressive social behavior. Each of these interventions is described below. Finally, we describe two comprehensive adolescent treatment programs that provide interventions that are appropriate to young people who are already using illicit drugs and who may already have abuse or dependence problems.

Mass Media

Possibly, drug abuse could be prevented by advertising in mass media, although only two studies have shown positive effects of such a strategy. In one of those studies, researchers at the University of Vermont compared the effects of a school-based prevention program with the effects of the school-based program plus a series of anti-smoking ads for preventing smoking. The students were in grades 4 through 6 when they received the intervention. The ads were developed using an extensive series of focus groups and youth surveys (Worden et al., 1988). The objectives of the ads were: (a) to show the advantages of not smoking and the disadvantages of smoking, (b) to demonstrate that most young people do not smoke, (c) to model the refusal of cigarettes, (d) to show that the tobacco industry wants kids to start smoking, and (e) to provide advice on quitting for those who already smoked. A diverse array of formats (e.g., situation comedy, cartoons, rock videos, and straightforward testimonials) were used in making ads in order to give the sense that they did not all come from the same source, but rather reflected general national norms. All ads were pilot tested, and new ads were created each year in this four-year campaign. Survey data were used to identify the most effective media channels and programs and time was purchased in order to ensure effective ad placement—a feature of anti-drug advertising that has often been missing.

Flynn and colleagues (Flynn, Worden, Secker-Walker, & Badger, 1992; Flynn, Worden, Secker-Walker, & Pirie, 1994; Flynn et al., 1997) describe the results of a large-scale study in which the school-based program was provided in two small media markets and the school-based program plus the media campaign was provided in two additional markets. Advertising had strong effects on adolescent smoking. After four years of intervention, the rate of smoking among students receiving both the school and media programs was 35% less than among those receiving only the school program (Flynn et al., 1992). These effects persisted through a two-year follow-up (Flynn et al., 1994). The program was also highly effective for youth identified to be at high risk of beginning smoking (Flynn et al., 1997). These results suggest that mass media could be effective in preventing smoking. Whether or not the prevention of smoking can contribute to the prevention of the abuse of other drugs is less clear.

Palmgreen, Donohew, Lorch, Hoyle, and Stephensen (2002) showed that a media campaign could prevent the onset of marijuana smoking. Like the Vermont group, Palmgreen et al. (in press) carefully developed a series of anti-marijuana ads. In addition, based on evidence that youths who are high in sensation seeking are at greatest risk to use drugs, they designed ads that were high in sensation value; that is, they were fast-paced, exciting, and attention getting in order to appeal to these young people. The prevalence of marijuana use began to decline in two communities when the campaign was introduced. The onset of the decline coincided with the time at which the campaign began, supporting the contention that the ads were responsible for the reduction in marijuana use. Whether the use that was prevented contributes to the prevention of abuse and dependence is still unknown.

Despite these positive effects, at least five other evaluations of media interventions on the use of substances did not find significant effects (Bauman, LaPrelle, Brown, Koch, & Padgett, 1991; See Flay, 2000). Thus, while media interventions show some promise, their efficacy is far from guaranteed.

Universal Interventions Directed at Parents

Evidence shows that parental monitoring and limit setting are related to the development of drug use and other problem behaviors (Ary, Duncan, Biglan et al., 1999; Ary, Duncan, Duncan et al., 1999; Dishion & Andrews, 1995). Therefore, it is reasonable to try to influence these parental practices. Although the efficacy of behavioral parenting skills programs for children and adolescents has been shown in numerous studies (Taylor & Biglan, 1998), most studies have not assessed whether these interventions contribute to the prevention of drug abuse.

In one important exception, Spoth and colleagues have been examining the value of family-focused interventions for the prevention of youth problem behaviors. These interventions are "universal" interventions in the sense that they target all families of middle school students. In one study, Spoth, Redmond, and Lepper (1999) assessed the value of the Iowa Strengthening Families Program for preventing alcohol use. This comprehensive program teaches skills to parents and children that are designed to improve discipline, communication, and family relations. Spoth, Redmond et al. (1999) found that the program led to significantly less alcohol use among teens one and two years after participation in the program when compared to teens who had been randomly assigned to a control group. Spoth's group also evaluated the effects of Preparing for the Drug Free Years (PDFY), a five session family-focused program that is designed to improve family communications and establish clear rules about the use of substances. Spoth, Reyes, Redmond, and Shin (1999) indicated that both PDFY and the Iowa Strengthening Families Program led to less initiation of the use of drugs. Moreover, PDFY delayed progression to higher levels of use among young people who had already initiated some drug use.

Comprehensive Community Interventions

Since a multiplicity of factors can contribute to drug use and abuse, comprehensive community interventions have been developed that are designed to: (a) implement school-based curricular interventions; (b) modify school policies relevant to (typically) tobacco and alcohol use; (c) mobilize parents to influence their children not to use tobacco, alcohol, and other drugs; (d) influence community organizations to engage in practices that would deter drug use; and (e) use media both to influence young people and to motivate activities of those who can influence young people. We summarize the results of three such programs here. Only one of them was designed to prevent illicit drug use, but all three bear on the efficacy of community interventions to affect substance use.

PROJECT NORTHLAND. This intervention (Perry, Williams, Forster, & Wolfson, 1993; Perry et al., 1996, 1998) was designed to prevent adolescent alcohol use. It tried to improve parent-child communication about alcohol use, enhance students' reasons for not using alcohol, strengthen students' beliefs that they were capable of resisting alcohol, reduce peer influences on drinking, improve alcohol use norms, and reduce students' ease of access to alcohol. The strategies used to accomplish these objectives were parental involvement and education, social-behavioral curricula delivered in the schools, peer leadership opportunities, and community-wide task force activities. The intervention was delivered to students in grades six through eight. Twenty school districts were randomly assigned to intervention or control conditions.

By the end of the 8th grade, compared with control students, intervention students reported significantly less alcohol use in the past week and in the past month, and reduced peer influence on behavior (Perry et al., 1996). The effects were stronger among students who had not previously tried alcohol. In addition, intervention students who were nonusers of alcohol at baseline reported significantly less cigarette and marijuana use. The intervention group also reported better attitudes and normative beliefs regarding alcohol use than did young people in comparison communities. However, by the 10th grade, the effects of the program on alcohol use had decayed (Perry et al., 1998).

THE MIDWESTERN PREVENTION PROJECT. This program is also known as Project STAR (Dwyer et al., 1989; Johnson et al. 1990; MacKinnon et al.,

1991; Pentz, Dwyer et al., 1989; Pentz, Johnson, Dwyer, & MacKinnon, 1989; Pentz, MacKinnon et al., 1989; Pentz, Trebow, Hansen, & MacKinnon, 1990). It is a comprehensive, multi-component, community-based program to reduce the prevalence of substance use among middle and junior high school students. The intervention included components targeting the school, media, parents, the community, and health policy. Goals of the program were: (a) to encourage young people to resist peer pressure to smoke and use drugs; (b) to prepare teens for the pressures involved in the transition to high school; (c) to counteract pro-smoking influences from adults, media, and the environment; and (d) to promote positive parent-child communication about substance prevention. The intervention began in the first year of middle school (6th or 7th grade). The school-based component included a 10-session curriculum teaching skills for resisting drugs and homework sessions with parents, and a five-session booster school program with more homework. Parent training and community organizing involved a series of planning meetings, annual educational seminars, and organizing efforts regarding drug prevention curricula and school policies. Mass media efforts included one- to two-minute news spots showing training and program implementation aired on the evening news by three major network stations, television and radio talk shows with project staff, press conferences, and articles describing baseline substance use and program goals.

Eight schools were matched on school characteristics and randomly assigned to either the intervention or a control condition. During interventions after the first and second year of the program, intervention students demonstrated a low rate of increase in smoking onset, while comparison students had a sharp increase in smoking onset (Pentz, Johnson et al., 1989; Pentz, MacKinnon et al., 1989). At the Year 3 evaluation, students in intervention schools reported significantly lower rates of tobacco and marijuana use, but not alcohol use, compared to students in control schools (Johnson et al., 1990). The greater the amount of program exposure teens received, the greater the changes in adolescent drug use behavior (Pentz et al., 1990). These findings underscore the importance of ensuring that school and intervention personnel deliver effective programs as intended—the poorer the quality of the delivery, the poorer the prevention effect.

PROJECT SIXTEEN.   Biglan, Ary, Duncan, Black, and Smolkowski (2000) report the evaluation of a comprehensive community intervention to prevent tobacco use. Sixteen pairs of small Oregon communities were randomly assigned to receive classroom-based prevention programs or the school-based program plus a community intervention. The school-based curriculum consisted of the grade 6–12 Programs to Advance Teen Health (PATH) curriculum, shown in an earlier study to reduce the rate of smoking among adolescents who reported cigarette use before the intervention (Ary et al., 1990). The community-based intervention consisted of five components: (a) media advocacy about the importance of preventing adolescent tobacco use, (b) youth anti-tobacco activities designed to involve young people in persuasive actions against tobacco use, (c) family communications about tobacco designed to expose children to their parents' opposition to their using tobacco, (d) a program of rewards for clerks for not selling tobacco to young people, and (e) implementation of cessation programs for minors cited for possession of tobacco.

Seventh and ninth grade students were surveyed annually for five years. The community program had significant effects on the prevalence of weekly cigarette use at Times 2 and 5 and the effect approached significance at Time 4. The intervention also affected the prevalence of smokeless tobacco among ninth grade boys at Time 2. Moreover, despite the fact that the intervention targeted only tobacco use, there was a significant effect on alcohol use among ninth graders; fewer young people in the community intervention communities reported using alcohol. Similarly, the intervention had a preventive effect on marijuana use. Significant effects were also reported for awareness of efforts to prevent illegal sales, attitudes toward tobacco, intentions to chew smokeless tobacco (males only), estimates of friends' smoking, and estimates of general peer deviance.

These results have important implications for preventing alcohol or marijuana use by preventing smoking. None of the intervention elements focused on alcohol or marijuana use, yet effects were found on the use of these substances. This could be because those who were prevented from smoking were less likely subsequently to use other substances. It could also be that the community intervention generally changed the norms for using any substance. Regardless of the reason, these results show that tobacco, alcohol, and drug use are all related in teens, both in their development and possibly in their prevention.

Interventions Focused on Aggressive Social Behavior of Children

As noted above, a subset of young people characterized by aggressive social behavior are at particularly high risk to develop substance abuse problems. Because these young people are also at risk for numerous other problems, including delinquency (Patterson et al., 1992) and high risk sexual behavior (Capaldi, Crosby, & Stoolmiller, 1996; Metzler, 1992; Metzler, Noell, Biglan, & Ary, 1994), a growing number of studies test strategies for preventing the development of problem behaviors among these young people. Some of these also assessed the effects of their interventions on smoking, alcohol, or drug use. We briefly review this literature here.

THE MONTREAL LONGITUDINAL-EXPERIMENTAL STUDY. This project evaluated the effects of parenting skills training and social skills training for
aggressive kindergarten boys (Tremblay, Pagani-Kurtz, Masse, & Vitaro,
1995). The boys were followed through age 15. Relative to boys randomly
assigned to a control group, fewer treated boys were held back or placed
in special classrooms. Treated boys reported significantly lower levels of
overall delinquency. Surprisingly, however, they did not differ from un-
treated boys when substance use (consuming alcohol, getting drunk, or
using marijuana) and vandalism were considered separately. Thus, the intervention contributed to a general lowering of problem behavior, but did
not clearly prevent substance use.

THE GOOD BEHAVIOR GAME. Kellam, Ling, Merisca, Brown, and
Ialongo (1998) reported on the effects of a classroom behavior management strategy called the Good Behavior Game on the aggressive behavior
of elementary school children. The game involves dividing the class into
teams that, as groups, receive rewards for periods of time in which they
meet standards for appropriate classroom behavior. At the outset of first
grade, 19 public elementary schools and their teachers were randomly assigned either to implement this program or not during first and second
grades. The game significantly reduced aggressive behavior in first grade.
Even in sixth grade, the effects of the program were detectable: teachers
rated boys who had received the Good Behavior Game in first grade as significantly less aggressive than boys in the control groups. The researchers
have not yet reported on whether the intervention was associated with reductions in illicit drug or alcohol use. However, they did find that boys who
had the intervention were significantly less likely to be smoking at age 14
(Kellam & Anthony, 1998).

LINKING THE INTERESTS OF FAMILIES AND TEACHERS (LIFT). Reid, Eddy,
Fetrow, and Stoolmiller (1999) described the evaluation of a 10-week intervention that included parent training, a classroom-based social skills
program, a program to reinforce appropriate social behavior on the playground, and arrangements designed to increase communication between
parents and children. First and fifth graders in 12 elementary schools were
randomly assigned either to receive or not to receive the program. At a
three-year follow-up, fifth graders who had been involved in the program
had a lower likelihood of a first arrest and less initiation of alcohol and marijuana use than did fifth graders not receiving the program (Eddy, Reid, &
Fetrow, 2000). These effects were found regardless of the level of problem
behavior initially exhibited by the children. First graders who received
LIFT were much less likely than comparison children to increase the level

of inattentive, impulsive, and hyperactive behavior over the follow-up period. Moreover, the rates of negative behavior in the playground setting were significantly lower among LIFT recipients compared to children in the control condition.

FAST TRACK.   The Fast Track prevention program (Conduct Problems Prevention Research Group, 1999a, 1999b) employs a set of comprehensive school-based services implemented between first and tenth grade to prevent the development of serious antisocial behavior in four sites across the United States selected from neighborhoods characterized by high crime and poverty. Specifically, all children in participating first grade classrooms receive teacher instruction using a structured curriculum that focuses on social problem solving, emotion recognition, friendship building, communication, and self-control skills. In addition, Fast Track staff offers additional interventions to "high-risk" children (selected based on high levels of teacher and parent reported aggressive and disruptive behavior at the end of kindergarten) and their parents. Additional interventions include parent-training groups focused on parenting skills and positive parent-school relationships, and social skills training and academic tutoring for the children. To promote participation in these weekend intervention groups, parents are paid for each session they attend, and staff provides transportation and childcare.

The only published results of Fast Track are from data collected after the first year of intervention. Possibly the most important findings relate to reductions in aggression in the high-risk sample because of the connections between early aggression and later aggression, and between aggression and drug use. Fast Track affected measures of aggression inconsistently, with some measures showing less aggression in the Fast Track children compared to controls, but other measures showing no differences. On a more positive note, high-risk Fast Track children exceeded high-risk control group children on a number of measures of social and academic competence. Similarly, parents of high-risk youngsters in the Fast Track schools showed evidence of better parenting and parent-school relationships on several measures. Whether these factors—together with more intervention in second grade—will lead to more impressive declines in child aggression will be important to assess as the study progresses, especially in light of the resource demands of this comprehensive program.

SCHOOLS AND HOMES IN PARTNERSHIP (SHIP).   Because children's aggressive behavior and reading difficulties during early elementary school years are risk factors for adolescent problem behaviors, this project evaluated the benefits of supplemental instruction in reading for children

with limited reading skill in grades K through 3 and parenting and social skills interventions for children with aggressive behavior problems
in these grades (Biglan et al., 2000). European-American and Hispanic
children from three communities who were selected for aggressiveness
or reading difficulties were randomly assigned to an intervention or no-
intervention control condition. Intervention families received parent training while their children received social skills training and supplementary
reading instruction over a two-year period. At the end of intervention, playground observations showed that treated children displayed less negative
social behavior than controls. At the end of a one-year follow-up, treated
children showed less teacher-rated depressed and anxious behavior and
less parent-rated coercive and antisocial behavior than controls. The study
provides further evidence that aggressive social behavior problems can be
ameliorated, but long-term follow-up will be needed to determine whether
these effects lead to reduced drug use and abuse.

Concluding Remarks: Multiple Strategies to Prevent Drug Abuse

Schools and communities that seek to reduce the prevalence of drug abuse
have multiple strategies available for doing so. Although none has been
definitively shown to prevent drug abuse, each has shown benefit in reducing drug use or in affecting aggressive social behavior—a well-established
precursor of drug abuse and a problem that is important to prevent in its
own right. Classroom-based curricular interventions that actively involve
young people in clarifying the norms against substance use and learning
skills for resisting social influence can have significant benefit in reducing
the proportion of young people who use tobacco, alcohol, and marijuana.
Although it has not been firmly established that preventing the use of
these substances will prevent the development of drug abuse, drug abuse
cannot develop among young people who do not use these substances.
Life Skills Training is the most extensively evaluated program of this type.
Effective implementation of it requires careful training and monitoring of
the integrity of its implementation.

Carefully developed ad campaigns targeting tobacco or marijuana use
hold the potential to reduce the use of these substances, although this is by
no means assured. However, since national campaigns targeting tobacco
and marijuana use are already underway (Kelder, Maibach, Worden,
Biglan, & Levitt, 2000), and considering the expense of developing an effective media campaign, individual communities may not need to implement
their own campaigns. Individual schools and communities can, however,
attempt to increase young people's attention to and involvement in the

media campaign by implementing activities that are consonant with it (Flay & Burton, 1990) such as local youth anti-drug activities (Biglan, Ary, Yudelson, Duncan, & Hood, 1996).

Evidence also suggests that comprehensive community campaigns that mobilize family, school, media, and community influences against substance use can have benefits over and above those provided by classroom-based interventions. However, thus far, highly experienced and well financed research groups have implemented the successful interventions. Communities that hope to duplicate these results will require a similar level of resources and expertise and careful monitoring of the interventions to ensure that they are implemented as designed. Furthermore, they should routinely collect data on the effectiveness of programs they implement to ensure that the program is working as it should.

Interventions designed to influence all parents in a community to engage in effective monitoring and limit setting can reach and influence a sufficient proportion of parents to have some impact on alcohol use (Spoth, Redmond et al., 1999). However, given the cost of these programs and the resources needed to recruit high-risk parents to participate in such programs, they may not be the optimal intervention for communities. Comparisons of "universal" interventions—such as Preparing for the Drug-Free Years—with those that target high-risk young people would clarify the relative merit of these two strategies.

We must also recognize that most prevention programs, even the best of them, have not evaluated their effects on drug abuse. Indeed, our most effective programs are unlikely to totally prevent drug abuse. As indicated earlier, drug-abusing teens are often involved in other problem behaviors such as delinquency and risky sexual behavior. Comprehensive community efforts to prevent drug use and abuse must also involve effective treatment for these teens, many of whom have come in contact with the juvenile justice system and are at risk for early and repeated incarceration.

Two programs with particular promise for these multi-problem youth are Multi-Dimensional Treatment Foster Family Care (Chamberlain, 1994), and Multisystemic Therapy (MST; Henggeler, Schoenwald, Borduin, Rowland, & Cunningham, 1998). Both principally target adolescents who have shown a pattern of repeated juvenile offending and are community-based alternatives to incarceration. Multi-Dimensional Treatment Foster Family Care intervention involves placing the adolescent in the home of a foster parent who has been extensively trained in behavior management skills and who implements specific plans to improve the adolescent's home and school performance while being continuously supported by an intervention staff. With multisystemic therapy, therapists plan an individualized treatment for each child based on: (a) the strengths and weaknesses of the child as well as members of the social systems in which the child operates (i.e., family, school, neighborhood, peer group); (b) empirical evidence that supports the use of particular strategies to address the particular strengths and weaknesses identified by the therapist; and (c) a set of guiding principles that describe MST generally (e.g., "Interventions target sequences of behavior within and between multiple systems that maintain the identified problem;" Henggeler et al., 1998, p. 23). Both programs have shown greater short- and long-term positive effects on delinquent behavior than alternative treatments (Borduin et al., 1995; Chamberlain & Reid, 1998), and both have preliminary evidence that they also reduce drug use (Henggeler et al., 1998). Furthermore, both appear to be cost-effective strategies (Aos, Phipps, Bamoski, & Lieb, 1999) for reducing delinquency and possibly drug abuse. Both also illustrate the kinds of intensive individualized strategies that may be necessary to reduce delinquency and drug abuse in multi-problem children, and highlight the need to prevent the development of these difficulties.

Finally, we recommend that communities implement evidence-based strategies to ameliorate aggressive behavior problems with children. Although these strategies have yet to be shown to prevent the development of drug abuse, aggressive behavior is so persistent and prognostic of such a wide array of problems in adolescents that interventions should be a high priority even if their impact on drug abuse proves to be limited.

References

American Psychiatric Association. (1994). *Diagnostic and statistical manual of mental disorders: DSM-IV* (4th ed.). Washington, DC: Author.

Aos, S., Phipps, P., Bamoski, R., & Lieb, R. (1999). *The comparative costs and benefits of programs to reduce crime: A review of national findings with implications for Washington State.* Olympia: Washington State Institute for Public Policy.

Ary, D.V., Biglan, A., Glasgow, R.E., Zoref, L., Black, C., Ochs, L.M., et al. (1990). The efficacy of social-influence prevention programs versus "standard care": Are new initiatives needed? *Journal of Behavioral Medicine, 13,* 281–296.

Ary, D.V., Duncan, T.E., Biglan, A., Metzler, C.W., Noell, J.W., & Smolkowski, K. (1999). Development of adolescent problem behavior. *Journal of Abnormal Child Psychology, 27,* 141–150.

Ary, D.V., Duncan, T.E., Duncan, S.C., & Hops, H. (1999). Adolescent problem behavior: The influence of parents and peers. *Behaviour Research & Therapy, 37,* 217–230.

Barrera, M., Jr., Biglan, A., Ary, D.V., & Li, F. (2001). Replication of a problem behavior model with American Indian, Hispanic, and Caucasian youth. *Journal of Early Adolescence, 21,* 133–157.

Bauman, K.E., & Ennett, S.T. (1996). On the importance of peer influence for adolescent drug use: Commonly neglected considerations. *Addiction, 91,* 185–198.

Bauman, K.E., LaPrelle, J., Brown, J.D., Koch, G.G., & Padgett, C.A. (1991). The influence of three mass media campaigns on variables related to adolescent cigarette smoking: Results of a field experiment. *American Journal of Public Health, 81,* 597–604.

Biglan, A., Ary, D.V., Duncan, T.E., Black, C., & Smolkowski, K. (2000). A randomized control trial of a community intervention to prevent adolescent tobacco use. *Tobacco Control, 9,* 12–24.

Biglan, A., Ary, D., Yudelson, H., Duncan, T.E., & Hood, D. (1996). Experimental evaluation of a modular approach to mobilizing antitobacco influences of peers and parents. *American Journal of Community Psychology, 24,* 311–339.

Biglan, A., Glasgow, R.E., Ary, D., & Thompson, R. (1987). How generalizable are the effects of smoking prevention programs? Refusal skills training and parent messages in a teacher-administered program. *Journal of Behavioral Medicine, 10,* 613–628.

Biglan, A., Severson, H., Ary, D.V., & Faller, C. (1987). Do smoking prevention programs really work? Attrition and the internal and external validity of an evaluation of a refusal skills training program. *Journal of Behavioral Medicine, 10,* 159–171.

Biglan, A., & Smolkowski, K. (2002). Intervention effects on adolescent drug use and critical influences on the development of problem behavior. In D.B. Kandel (Ed.), *Stages and pathways of drug involvement: Examining the gateway hypothesis.* New York: Cambridge University Press.

Borduin, C.M., Mann, B.J., Cone, L.T., Henggeler, S.W., Fucci, B.R., Blaske, D.M., et al. (1995). Multisystemic treatment of serious juvenile offenders: Long-term prevention of criminality and violence. *Journal of Consulting & Clinical Psychology, 63,* 569–578.

Botvin, G.J. (2000). Preventing drug abuse in schools: Social and competence enhancement approaches targeting individual-level etiologic factors. *Addictive Behaviors, 25,* 887–897.

Botvin, G.J., Baker, E., Filazzola, A.D., & Botvin, E.M. (1990). A cognitive-behavioral approach to substance abuse prevention: One-year follow-up. *Addictive Behaviors, 15,* 47–63.

Botvin, G.J., Epstein, J.A., Baker, E., Diaz, T., & Ifill-Williams, M. (1997). School-based drug abuse prevention with inner-city minority youth. *Journal of Child & Adolescent Substance Abuse, 6,* 5–19.

Capaldi, D.M., Crosby, L., & Stoolmiller, M. (1996). Predicting the timing of first sexual intercourse for at-risk adolescent males. *Child Development, 67,* 344–359.

Chamberlain, P. (1994). *Family connections: Treatment foster care for adolescents with delinquency.* Eugene, OR: Castalia.

Chamberlain, P., & Reid, J.B. (1998). Comparison of two community alternatives to incarceration for chronic juvenile offenders. *Journal of Consulting & Clinical Psychology, 66,* 624–633.

Cohen, M. (1998). The monetary value of saving a high-risk youth. *Journal of Quantitative Criminology, 14,* 5–33.

Conduct Problems Prevention Research Group. (1999a). Initial impact of the fast track prevention trial for conduct problems: I. The high-risk sample. *Journal of Consulting & Clinical Psychology, 67,* 631–647.

Conduct Problems Prevention Research Group. (1999b). Initial impact of the fast track prevention trial for conduct problems: II. Classroom effects. *Journal of Consulting & Clinical Psychology, 67,* 648–657.

Dishion, T.J., & Andrews, D.W. (1995). Preventing escalation in problem behaviors with high-risk young adolescents: Immediate and 1-year outcomes. *Journal of Consulting & Clinical Psychology, 63,* 538–548.

Dishion, T.J., Capaldi, D., Spracklen, K.M., & Li, F. (1995). Peer ecology of male adolescent drug use [Special issue]. *Development & Psychopathology, 7,* 803–824.

Dishion, T.J., Eddy, M., Haas, E., & Li, F. (1997). Friendships and violent behavior during adolescence. *Social Development, 6,* 207–223.

Dishion, T.J., Spracklen, K.M., Andrews, D.W., & Patterson, G.R. (1996). Deviancy training in male adolescents friendships. *Behavior Therapy, 27,* 373–390.

Donaldson, S.I., Graham, J.W., Piccinin, A.M., & Hansen, W.B. (1995). Resistance-skills training and onset of alcohol use: Evidence for beneficial and potentially harmful effects in public schools and in private Catholic schools. *Health Psychology, 14*, 291–300.

Dwyer, J.H., MacKinnon, D.P., Pentz, M.A., Flay, B.R., Hansen, W.B., Wang, E.Y., et al. (1989). Estimating intervention effects in longitudinal studies. *American Journal of Epidemiology, 130*, 781–795.

Eddy, J.M., Reid, J.B., & Fetrow, R.A. (2000). An elementary school-based prevention program targeting modifiable antecedents of youth delinquency and violence: Linking interests of families and teachers (LIFT). *Journal of Emotional & Behavioral Disorders, 8*, 165–186.

Ennett, S.T., Tobler, N.S., Ringwalt, C.L., & Flewelling, R.L. (1994). How effective is drug abuse resistance education? A meta-analysis of Project DARE outcome evaluations. *American Journal of Public Health, 84*, 1394–1401.

Flay, B.R. (2000). Approaches to substance use prevention utilizing school curriculum plus social environment change. *Addictive Behaviors, 25*, 861–885.

Flay, B.R., & Burton, D. (1990). Effective mass communication strategies for health campaigns. In C. Atkin & L. Wallack (Eds.), *Mass communication and public health* (pp. 129–146). Newbury Park, CA: Sage.

Flynn, B.S., Worden, J.K., Secker-Walker, R.H., & Badger, G.J. (1992). Prevention of cigarette smoking through mass media intervention and school programs. *American Journal of Public Health, 82*, 827–834.

Flynn, B.S., Worden, J.K., Secker-Walker, R.H., & Pirie, P.L. (1994). Mass media and school interventions for cigarette smoking prevention: Effects 2 years after completion. *American Journal of Public Health, 84*, 1148–1150.

Flynn, B.S., Worden, J.K., Secker-Walker, R.H., Pirie, P.L., Badger, G.J., & Carpenter, J.H. (1997). Long-term responses of higher and lower risk youths to smoking prevention interventions. *Preventive Medicine, 26*, 389–394.

Glantz, M.D., Weinberg, N.Z., Miner, L.L., & Colliver, J.D. (1999). The etiology of drug abuse: Mapping the paths. In M.D. Glantz & C.R. Hartel (Eds.), *Drug abuse: Origins & interventions* (pp. 3–45). Washington, DC: American Psychological Association.

Goeders, N.E. (1998). Stress, the hypothalamic-pituitary-adrenal axis, and vulnerability to drug abuse. *NIDA Research Monograph, 169*, 83–104.

Henggeler, S.W., Schoenwald, S.K., Borduin, C.M., Rowland, M.D., & Cunningham, P.B. (1998). *Multisystemic treatment of antisocial behavior in children and adolescents.* New York: Guilford Press.

Institute of Medicine. (1996). *Pathways of addiction: Opportunities in drug abuse research.* Washington, DC: National Academy Press.

Johnson, C.A., Pentz, M.A., Weber, M.D., Dwyer, J.H., Baer, N., MacKinnon, D.P., et al. (1990). Relative effectiveness of comprehensive community programming for drug abuse prevention with high-risk & low-risk adolescents. *Journal of Consulting & Clinical Psychology, 58*, 447–456.

Kandel, D.B., Yamaguchi, K., & Chen, K. (1992). Stages of progression in drug involvement from adolescence to adulthood: Further evidence for the gateway theory. *Journal of Studies on Alcohol, 53*, 447–457.

Kelder, S.H., Maibach, E., Worden, J.K., Biglan, A., & Levitt, A. (2000). Planning and initiation of the ONDCP National Youth Anti-Drug Media Campaign. *Journal of Public Health Management and Practice, 6(3)*, 14–26.

Kellam, S.G., & Anthony, J.C. (1998). Targeting early antecedents to prevent tobacco smoking: Findings from an epidemiologically based randomized field trial. *American Journal of Public Health, 88*, 1490–1495.

Kellam, S.G., Ling, X., Merisca, R., Brown, C.H., & Ialongo, N. (1998). The effect of the level of aggression in the first grade classroom on the course and malleability of aggressive behavior into middle school. *Development & Psychopathology, 10*, 165–185.

MacKinnon, D.P., Johnson, C.A., Pentz, M.A., Dwyer, J.H., Hansen, W.B., Flay, B.R., Wang E.Y.I. (1991). Mediating mechanisms in a school-based drug prevention program: First-year effects of the Midwestern Prevention Project. *Health Psychology, 10*, 164–172.

Metzler, C.W. (1992). The validation of a construct of high-risk sexual behavior in heterosexual adolescents. *Journal of Adolescent Research, 7*, 233–249.

Metzler, C.W., Noell, J., Biglan, A., & Ary, D. (1994). The social context for risky sexual behavior among adolescents. *Journal of Behavioral Medicine, 17*, 419–438.

Monitoring the Future. (1999). *Trends in annual and 30-Day prevalence of use of various drugs for 8th, 10th, 12th Graders, 1991–99.* Retrieved October 11, 2000, from http: // monitoringthefuture.org / data / 99data.html

Palmgreen, P., Donohew, L., Lorch, E.P., Hoyle, R.H., & Stephensen, M.T. (2002). Television campaigns and sensation seeking targeting of adolescent marijuana use: A controlled time-series approach. In R.C. Hornik (Ed.), *Public health communication: Evidence for behavior change* (pp. 35–56). Hillsdale, NJ: Erlbaum.

Patterson, G.R. (1999). A proposal relating a theory of delinquency to societal rates of juvenile crime: Putting Humpty Dumpty together again. In M.J. Cox & J. Brooks-Gunn (Eds.), *Conflict and cohesion in families: Causes and consequences* (pp. 11–35). Mahwah, NJ: Lawrence Erlbaum.

Patterson, G.R., DeBaryshe, B.D., & Ramsey, E. (1989). A developmental perspective on anti-social behavior [Special issue]. *American Psychologist, 44*, 329–335.

Patterson, G.R., Dishion, T.J., & Yoerger, K. (2000). Adolescent growth in new forms of problem behavior: Macro- and micro-peer dynamics. *Prevention Science, 1*, 3–13.

Patterson, G.R., Forgatch, M.S., Yoerger, K.L., & Stoolmiller, M. (1998). Variables that initiate and maintain an early-onset trajectory for juvenile offending. *Development & Psychopathology, 10*, 531–547.

Patterson, G.R., Reid, J.B., & Dishion, T.J. (1992). *Antisocial boys: A social interactional approach* (Vol. 4). Eugene, OR: Castalia.

Patterson, G.R., & Yoerger, K. (1999). Intraindividual growth in covert antisocial behaviour: A necessary precursor to chronic juvenile and adult arrests? *Criminal Behaviour and Mental Health, 9(1)*, 24–38.

Pentz, M.A., Dwyer, J.H., MacKinnon, D.P., Flay, B.R., Hansen, W.B., Wang, E.Y., et al. (1989). A multicommunity trial for primary prevention of adolescent drug abuse. Effects on drug use prevalence. *Journal of the American Medical Association, 261*, 3259–3266.

Pentz, M.A., Johnson, C.A., Dwyer, J.H., & MacKinnon, D.M. (1989). A comprehensive community approach to adolescent drug abuse prevention: Effects on cardiovascular disease risk behaviors. *Annals of Medicine, 21*, 219–222.

Pentz, M.A., MacKinnon, D.P., Dwyer, J.H., Wang, E.Y., Hansen, W.B., Flay, B.R., et al. (1989). Longitudinal effects of the Midwestern Prevention Project on regular and experimental smoking in adolescents. *Preventive Medicine, 18*, 304–321.

Pentz, M.A., Trebow, E.A., Hansen, W.B., & MacKinnon, D.P. (1990). Effects of program implementation on adolescent drug use behavior: The Midwestern Prevention Project (MPP). *Evaluation Review, 14*, 264–289.

Perry, C.L., Williams, C.L., Forster, J.L., & Wolfson, M. (1993). Background, conceptualization and design of a community-wide research program on adolescent alcohol use: Project Northland. *Health Education Research, 8*, 125–136.

Perry, C.L., Williams, C.L., Komro, K.A., Veblen-Mortenson, S., Forster, J.L., Bernstein-Lachter, R., et al. (1998, February). *Project Northland—Phase II: Community action to reduce adolescent alcohol use.* Paper presented at the Fourth Symposium on Community Action Research and the Prevention of Alcohol and other Drug Problems: A Kettil Bruun Society Thematic Meeting, Russell, New Zealand.

Perry, C.L., Williams, C.L., Veblen-Mortenson, S., Toomey, T.L., Komro, K.A., Anstine, P.S., et al. (1996). Project Northland: Outcomes of a community-wide alcohol use prevention program during early adolescence. *American Journal of Public Health, 86,* 956–965.

Reid, J.B., Eddy, J.M., Fetrow, R.A., & Stoolmiller, M. (1999). Description and immediate impacts of a preventive intervention for conduct problems [Special issue]. *American Journal of Community Psychology, 27,* 483–517.

Rice, D.P., Kelman, S., Miller, L.S., & Dunmeyer, S. (1990). *The economic costs of alcohol and drug abuse and mental illness: 1985.* San Francisco: University of California, Institute for Health & Aging.

Robins, L.N., & McEvoy, L. (1990). Conduct problems as predictors of substance abuse. In L.N. Robins & M. Rutter (Eds.), *Straight and devious pathways from childhood to adulthood* (pp. 182–204). Cambridge, MA: Cambridge University Press.

Spoth, R., Redmond, C., & Lepper, H. (1999). Alcohol initiation outcomes of universal family-focused preventive interventions: One- and two-year follow-ups of a controlled study [Special issue]. *Journal of Studies on Alcohol Supplement, 13,* 103–111.

Spoth, R., Reyes, M.L., Redmond, C., & Shin, C. (1999). Assessing a public health approach to delay onset and progression of adolescent substance use: Latent transition and log-linear analyses of longitudinal family preventive intervention outcomes. *Journal of Consulting & Clinical Psychology, 67,* 619–630.

Substance Abuse & Mental Health Services Administration. (1995). *National Household Survey on Drug Abuse: Population estimates 1994.* Washington, DC: U.S. Department of Health and Human Services.

Taylor, T.K., & Biglan, A. (1998). Behavioral family interventions: A review for clinicians and policymakers. *Clinical Child and Family Psychology Review, 1(1),* 41–60.

Tobler, N.S., Lessard, T., Marshall, D., Ochshorn, P., & Roona, M. (1999). Effectiveness of school-based drug prevention programs for marijuana use. *School Psychology International, 20(1),* 105–37.

Tobler, N.S., Roona, M.R., Ochshorn, P., Marshall, D.G., Streke, A.V., & Stackpole, K.M. (2000). School-based adolescent drug prevention programs: 1998 meta-analysis. *Journal of Primary Prevention, 20,* 275–336.

Tremblay, R.E., Pagani-Kurtz, L., Masse, L.C., & Vitaro, F. (1995). A bimodal preventive intervention for disruptive kindergarten boys: Its impact through mid-adolescence. *Journal of Consulting & Clinical Psychology, 63,* 560–568.

Walker, H.M., Colvin, G., & Ramsey, E. (1995). *Antisocial behavior in school: Strategies and best practices.* Pacific Grove, CA: Brooks/Cole.

Worden, J.K., Flynn, B.S., Geller, B.M., Chen, M., Shelton, L.G., Secker-Walker, R.H., et al. (1988). Development of a smoking prevention mass media program using diagnostic and formative research. *Preventive Medicine, 17,* 531–558.

Chapter 5

Sexual Risk Behaviors among Adolescents

Henry D. Anaya, Susan M. Cantwell,
and Mary Jane Rotheram-Borus

Patterns of sexual behaviors are complex and culturally specific and the average age of sexual initiation and its consequences vary worldwide (Werdelin, Misfeldt, Melbye, & Olsen, 1995). These cultural and developmental factors relate directly to the negative consequences that occur from unprotected adolescent sex: high rates of teenage pregnancy, STDs, abortion, and HIV infection.

Adolescents participating in risky sexual behaviors often participate in other risky behaviors—using alcohol and drugs, dropping out of school, having contact with the juvenile justice system, etc. The adoption of these multiple problem behaviors often lead to youth becoming unemployable adults (Donovan, Jessor & Costa, 1991; Jessor & Jessor, 1977; Koniak-Griffin & Brecht, 1995). Multiple problem behaviors are more likely among specific adolescent subgroups (e.g., runaway, homeless, and gay youth) and among adolescents from dysfunctional families or who have been victimized or are disconnected from their parents (see, for example, Booth, Zhang, & Kwiatkowski, 1999; Remafedi, 1994; Rotheram-Borus et al., 1992). In response to this risk, a large number of prevention programs (n = 36) have been effective in reducing sexual risk acts (see Jemmott & Jemmott, 2000; Kirby, 2000 for reviews). Eight types of community-level approaches have been found effective.

This chapter summarizes the research data describing adolescent sexuality and its consequences, presents policy issues regarding adolescent sexual health, and discusses some programs that have successfully reduced adolescents' high-risk sexual behaviors. This information is presented in six sections: 1) patterns of risk, 2) consequences of sexual activity, 3) associations of sexual risk to multiple problem behaviors, 4) high-risk subpopulations, 5) factors mediating sexual risk, and 6) effective intervention approaches.

This chapter aims to challenge readers to think broadly about the issue of adolescent sexual behavior. Toward this end, the final section will link these adolescent activities to social-psychological theories that help to explain why adolescents, in particular, are prone to engaging in sexually risky behaviors.

Patterns of Risk

High-risk sexual behaviors include sexual experiences before 17–18 years of age, sexual intercourse unprotected by condoms, having multiple sex partners, bartering sex (e.g., for drugs or money), sexual intercourse with partners with known risk factors (i.e., HIV+ partners, injecting drug users, sex workers) and sexual encounters in the context of alcohol and drug use. Youth who engage in such activities place themselves at higher risk than their peers for contracting HIV, other STDs, and becoming pregnant (Breakwell, Millward, & Fife-Schaw, 1994; Rotheram-Borus & Gwadz, 1993). Youth at particularly high risk include those who are: 1) homeless or runaway; 2) self-identified as gay; 3) incarcerated; 4) psychiatrically disturbed, or 5) live in inner city areas where drug dealing is high (Rotheram-Borus & Gwadz, 1993).

While the age of sexual initiation varies throughout the world, for most people it occurs during their teenage years (ages 16–19; UNAIDS/WHO, 1998b). For example, by 15 years of age, 53% of young people in Greenland, 38% of young people in Denmark (Werdelin et al., 1995), and 69% of young people in Sweden (Klanger, Tyden, & Ruusuvaara, 1993) have experienced intercourse. The median age of initiation in England is 17 years (Wellings et al., 1995), 16 years in the United States (Zelnik & Shah, 1983), and 16.8 years in Sweden (Schwartz, 1993). These variations in age of sexual initiation indicate that we cannot generalize about a starting point for young people's introduction to sexual activity (Cleland & Ferry, 1995).

In the United States, epidemiological evidence shows that more than three-fourths of American adolescents have sexual intercourse by the age of nineteen (Centers for Disease Control and Prevention [CDC], 1991; Hatcher et al., 1994) and recent trends suggest that American youth are initiating sexual activity at progressively younger ages (Alan Guttmacher Institute,

1994; CDC, 2000e). By the age of 16, 42% of teens have had sexual intercourse and this figure rises to about 80% by age 18 years (Alan Guttmacher Institute, 1994; Anderson, Koniak-Griffin, & Keenan, 1999), with a small minority (7.2%) having their first sexual experience before the age of thirteen (CDC, 1999b). Over a third of all U.S. adolescents (34.8%) are currently sexually active (having sexual intercourse during the preceding 3 months), and about one in six (16.6%) has had four or more sex partners (CDC, 1999b).

There are both racial/ethnic and gender differences in early sexual activity. African American male and female students are more likely than Hispanic and White students to: 1) have engaged in sexual intercourse; 2) initiate sexual intercourse before age 13; and 3) be currently sexually active (CDC, 2000e). Concerning gender, male students (12.2%) are significantly more likely than female students (4.4%) to initiate sexual intercourse before the age of 13 (CDC, 2000e). This significant gender difference is present for all racial/ethnic subpopulations, and students in grades 9, 10, and 12.

One of the consequences of early sexual activity is the finding that teens who are sexually active during early adolescence are more likely to have unprotected sex (Pratt, Mosher, Bachrach, & Horn, 1984; Taylor, Kagay, & Leichenko, 1986). The risk posed by unprotected sex is reflected in adolescents' disproportionately higher rates of STD infection and unwanted pregnancies compared to adults (Braverman & Strasburger, 1994; Maxwell, Bastani & Yan, 1995). Nationwide, among adolescents who are currently sexually active, 42% report not using condoms during last sexual intercourse (CDC, 1999f). The proportion of students who use condoms decreases with grade level, from a high of 67% of 9th grade students to 48% of 12th graders (CDC, 1999f). Males (65.5%) are significantly more likely than females (50.7%), and African Americans (70%) are significantly more likely than Hispanics or Whites (55.2% and 55% respectively) to report condom use (CDC, 2000e).

The problems of early sexual initiation and unprotected sex are compounded when adolescents also have many sexual partners. Researchers have found racial/ethnic and gender differences in terms of multiple sex partners. Having multiple sex partners is more common among male students (19.3%) than female (13.1%). Also, more African American (48.1%) and Hispanic (23.0%) male students have multiple partners than Caucasian male students (12.1%; CDC, 2000e).

The activity of bartering sex (e.g., for drugs, money, food) is also known as "survival sex." Survival sex is most commonly practiced by runaway and homeless youth, and will be discussed in greater detail in the section on high-risk populations.

Sexual intercourse with a partner with known risk factors is of great concern to researchers. Recent data indicates that at least a third of HIV-positive adolescents are likely to continue their risky behaviors after learning of their serostatus (Hein, Dell, Futterman, Rotheram-Borus, & Shaffer, 1995; Rotheram-Borus et al., 1997). A possible solution to this problem is a simple screening of partners; the implication being that by screening, sex with high-risk partners could be avoided or the risk minimized by the use of safe-sex practices (Rotheram-Borus & Koopman, 1991). The problem with this strategy is that people lie in order to engage in sex (Keeling, 1988). Also, otherwise good judgment can be clouded and inhibitions relaxed if alcohol and drugs are used (Crowe & George, 1989).

A number of studies have documented a relationship between risky sexual behavior and substance use among adolescents (see Koniak-Griffin & Brecht, 1995). This issue will be discussed further in the section on associations of sexual risk to multiple problem behaviors.

Consequences of Sexual Activity

Early and unprotected sex places teens at risk for a variety of negative outcomes. Together these behaviors considerably increase the risk of getting (or making someone) pregnant and of contracting and spreading STDs—including HIV. In order to develop programs that promote safe sex among adolescents, researchers must understand how these high-risk behaviors evolve throughout the processes of adolescent development and within a distinct adolescent culture.

Teenage Pregnancy

Teenage pregnancy rates in the United States are much higher than those of many other developed countries (Singh & Darroch, 2000). Recent evidence suggests that the rate of pregnancy has declined for all women less than 30-years-old, with the sharpest drop occurring among adolescents (CDC/NCHS, 2000c). Despite these declining rates, about one in eight young women aged 15 to 19 years becomes pregnant each year (approximately 900,000), a figure that has changed little since the late 1970s (CDC, 1999d; CDC/NCHS, 2000c; Hatcher et al., 1994). While less than 10% of all adolescents become pregnant, this reflects a rate of about one in four sexually active adolescents. Most (about 78%) of these teen pregnancies are unintended and about one in four of them end in abortion (CDC/NCHS, 2000c). Nationally, only 6.3% of high school students report being pregnant or having gotten someone pregnant (CDC, 2000e). As expected, both self-report and official estimates indicate that pregnancy rates among adolescents increase with age (CDC, 2000e; CDC/NCHS, 2000c). For example, 13.8% of female students in grade 12 reported that they have been pregnant, which was significantly higher than those in lower grades (CDC, 2000e). Racial/ethnic differences are also found in teen pregnancy. For example, although African-American women report that they want approximately the same number of births as White women do, the adolescent birth rate is more than twice as high among them as compared to Whites, and birth rates for Hispanics are higher still (CDC, 2000e).

In 1999, only 16% of sexually active high school students were using birth control pills at the time of last sexual intercourse, as compared to 21% in 1991 (CDC, 1999c; CDC, 2000e). The overall use of birth control pills has been shown to increase with grade level (CDC, 2000e); racial/ethnic differences have also been found in the use of birth control pills, with Caucasian students (21%) significantly more likely to use them than Hispanic and African-American students (7.8% and 7.7% respectively; CDC, 2000e).

Teen Parenthood

Although teenage birth rates have declined between 1991 and 1998 by approximately 18%, the rates are still higher than or similar to rates found in the early to mid-1980s (Ventura, Curtin, & Mathews, 2000). Although the birth rate among 15–19 year olds has been steadily decreasing for over 40 years, the number of births that have occurred to unmarried women 15–19 years of age has risen dramatically during the same period (CDC 2000d).[1] Currently, about three in 10 children are born to unmarried adolescents, although this is a significant decrease from approximately five out of 10 births in the 1970s (Hollander, 1996). Decreased premarital sexual activity, increased condom use, and the use of implant and injectable contraceptives may account for these declines and provide implications for intervention strategies (Ventura et al., 2000). High birth rates, like high pregnancy rates, are associated with low socioeconomic status (SES), and thus, more likely among disenfranchised minorities (Jemmott & Jemmott, 1996). Substantial evidence indicates that school-age mothers complete less schooling (Hayes, 1987; Hofferth & Moore, 1979), and are more likely to experience divorce (Moore & Waite, 1981). These two factors, combined with higher rates of non-marital childbearing, result in women being more likely to

---

1 These data are not inconsistent, in that the rate is defined as the number of births to a group of 1,000 teenagers. Both the birth rate (the proportion of teens giving birth) and the number of teen women in the population affect the number of births attributed to teenagers. Therefore, trends in the birth rate and the number of births will not necessarily be the same.

be single heads of economically challenged families (Berry, Shillington, Peak, & Hohman, 2000).

Abortion

Although African Americans and Hispanics have twice the pregnancy rates of Caucasians, pregnancies among African-American women are twice as likely to end in abortion as pregnancies among White and Hispanic women (CDC, 2000c). Furthermore, there are wide variations in abortion access. For some, especially those in rural areas, abortion clinics may not be available within several hundred miles. For example, one study estimated that 27% of non-hospital patients in the United States traveled at least 50 miles from their homes to reach an abortion clinic; 18% traveled 50–100 miles, and 9% traveled over 100 miles (Henshaw, 1991).

Sexually Transmitted Diseases

STDs (e.g., herpes, gonorrhea, syphilis, and chancroid) have been described as the most destructive infectious diseases affecting adolescents (Cates, 1990), with young people under 25 years of age accounting for about two-thirds of an annual estimate of 12 million STD cases in the United States (CDC, 1999e). Annually, about three million cases of STDs occur among U.S. teenagers (CDC, 1998b). Adolescents are at higher risk than adults for contracting STDs (Braverman & Strasburger, 1994), and there are various reasons for this. They are more likely to: 1) have multiple sexual partners and shorter-term relationships; 2) engage in unprotected sex; and 3) have partners who are at higher risk for STDs (CDC, 1999g; Gittes & Irwin, 1993). STD infection also increases the chances of HIV infection, given that the acquisition and transmission routes of both are similar (Mezzich et al., 1997). Recent evidence also suggests that female adolescents may be especially vulnerable to STDs and HIV due to incomplete maturation (Mezzich et al., 1997).

The incidence of STDs varies by race/ethnicity, and STDs are substantially more common among African Americans than among Whites. For example, in 1994, the gonorrhea rates among African-American male and female adolescents 15 to 19 years of age were, on average, more than 28 times higher than those among White teens of the same age range (Jemmott & Jemmott, 1996).

HIV/AIDS Among Young People.   Globally, at least ten million young people aged 10–24 years are living with HIV or AIDS, accounting for about one-third of the total number of infections (UNAIDS/WHO,

1998c). About 7,000 10–24 year olds (or five persons every minute) are infected daily (UNAIDS/WHO, 1998a). National monitoring of HIV infection among adolescents is not yet available in the United States. However, based on current estimates of HIV infection among young persons (0.32%; McQuillan, Khare, Kareon, Schable & Vlahov, 1997) and a series of seroprevalence studies in high-risk subgroups, it has been estimated that 112,000 American youth are currently infected with HIV (Rotheram-Borus, O'Keefe, Kracker, & Foo, 2000). Youth aged 15–24 years represent about half of the newly acquired HIV infections in the United States (UNAIDS/WHO, 1998a), and in 1998, 1,798 young people aged 13 to 24 years were diagnosed with AIDS, bringing a total of 27,860 AIDS cases in this age group (CDC, 1999e). The national decline of AIDS incidence has not been accompanied by a decline in the number of new HIV cases among youth (CDC, 1998a), and young people continue to be vulnerable to the epidemic. AIDS among 15–24 year olds is the seventh most common cause of death (Hoyert, Kochanek, & Murphy, 1999), and African-American youth are particularly affected. In the United States, African-Americans account for 56% of all HIV cases reported in the 13–24 age group (CDC, 1999e), and among African Americans aged 25–44, AIDS is the leading cause of death (National Center for Health Statistics, 2000).

The majority of young people in the United States (approximately 58%) who are infected with HIV contract the infection through sexual transmission (CDC, 1998a; 1999e). In the 13- to 24-year age range, 51% of all AIDS cases reported among males in 1998 were among men who have sex with men (MSM); 10% were among injection drug users (IDUs); and 9% were among young men infected heterosexually (CDC, 1999e).

Young women infected with HIV are at risk for transmitting to their children (UNAIDS/WHO, 1998a). In the early 1990s, before the advent of prenatal preventive treatments, between 1,000 and 2,000 infants were born with HIV infection each year in the U.S. Between 1992 and 1998, perinatally acquired AIDS cases in the U.S. declined 75% due to broad HIV counseling and testing and availability of highly active antiretroviral therapies (CDC, 1999a).

Associations of Sexual Risk to Multiple Problem Behaviors

Sexual risk behavior has been shown to be associated with substance use, school dropout, juvenile delinquency, and unemployment (Mott & Haurin, 1988). Youth tend to engage in a cluster of negative or risky behaviors (Jessor & Jessor, 1977). Recent research has broadened the descriptive approach of the theory of problem behaviors to a social, ecological approach that seeks to understand the dynamic relationship among these behaviors.

Substance Use

Substance use is consistently shown to be associated with high-risk sexual activity (Elliott & Morse, 1989, Hingson, Strunin, Berlin & Heeren, 1990; Jemmott & Jemmott, 1993, Strunin & Hingson, 1992), and is also shown to be both directly and indirectly associated with an increased risk for acquiring HIV, as well as a number of STDs (Mezzich et al., 1997). Nationally, about one-fourth (24.8%) of sexually active students used alcohol or drugs at last sexual intercourse; this behavior is more common among male students than female students (CDC, 2000e). Only 2% of high school students report having injected an illegal drug (CDC, 1999e). Drug injection led to 6% of HIV diagnoses reported among those aged 13–14 years between January 1994 and June 1997 in 25 states (CDC, 1998a). Compared to non-drug using peers, female adolescent drug users tend to have older friends (Stattin & Magnusson, 1990) and boyfriends (Stattin & Magnusson, 1990). Female adolescent drug users also initiate sexual intercourse at an earlier age, have intercourse more frequently, are less likely to use condoms, and are more likely to have abortions (Rosenbaum & Kandel, 1990; Vaglum & Vaglum, 1987).

Delinquency

Delinquency and substance use tend to precede sexual involvement (Elliott & Morse, 1989). Melchert and Burnett (1990) show significant differences in sexual risk behaviors between incarcerated and non-incarcerated youth. Incarcerated youth were significantly more likely to have initiated sexual activity at an earlier age, had unreliable use of contraceptives, and were more likely to have higher rates of pregnancy.

School Dropout

Out-of-school youth (who have been estimated to be 11% of all school-age adolescents; National Center for Education Statistics, 1998) are particularly prone to participating in high-risk sexual behavior. About 70% of dropouts (aged 14–19 years) are sexually active (compared to 45% of in-school youth), and a significantly higher percentage of dropouts (36.4%) report having four or more sexual partners than in-school youth (14%; CDC, 1994).

Unemployment

Few researchers have linked macroeconomic issues such as community influence and unemployment to the sexual behaviors of young adolescents, although numerous hypotheses have been developed (Ku, Sonenstein, & Pleck, 1993). Ongoing studies of social capital and social disintegration may soon provide evidence of these processes. One area of inquiry examines how young men's employment and economic opportunities affect issues such as sexual behavior and partnership formation. Wilson (1987) hypothesizes that a central tenet of increasing rates of non-marital childbearing among African-American women was the declining employment opportunities of African-American men. For example, researchers found that young men in areas with high unemployment have more sexual partners and are more likely to have made a partner pregnant than those in neighborhoods with higher employment (Ku et al., 1993).

Youth with Mental Health Problems

Psychological distress has been linked to risky sexual behavior through stress-related depression (Rotheram-Borus, Koopman, & Bradley, 1989), low self-esteem, and low contraceptive use (Hayes, 1987). A reduction in mental health symptoms (e.g., alcohol/drug misuse, suicidality, and depression) over time is effective in preventing AIDS-related risk behaviors (i.e., IV drug use, prostitution, and choice of risky partners) in adolescents (Stiffman, Dore, Earls, & Cunningham, 1992).

High-Risk Subpopulations

Most youth do not run away from home, barter sex, partner with injecting drug users, or become incarcerated. For example, it has been estimated that fewer than 2% of adolescents run away from home (Zide & Cherry, 1992) and approximately 3% of high school students partner with injecting drug users (Hingson et al., 1990). However, for the small proportion of youths who do engage in these types of behaviors, the chances that they will engage in risky sexual behaviors are high. Runaway and homeless youth (Rotheram-Borus, Mahler, Koopman, & Langabeer, 1996), gay youth (Remafedi, 1994), those who are incarcerated (DiClemente, Lanier, Horan, & Lodico, 1991), psychiatrically disturbed (DiClemente, Ponton, Hartley, & McKenna, 1989), or live in inner cities (Keller et al., 1991), have high rates of sexual risk acts. In addition, these at-risk youth are found to be more sexually active 3 to 5 years earlier than their peers (Rotheram-Borus

& Gwadz, 1993). For example, runaways have their first sexual contact at a mean age of 12.5 years, gay males at 12.7 years (Rotheram-Borus et al., 1992), and psychiatrically disturbed youths at 10.7 years (DiClemente et al., 1989).

Runaway/Homeless Youth

Risky sexual behaviors are common among runaways and homeless youth. These youth tend to have multiple sexual partners, use condoms infrequently, and engage in survival sex (i.e., exchanging sex for money, drugs, clothes, food, or a bed; Robertson, 1989; Rotheram-Borus et al., 1992, 1996; Yates, Mackenzie, Pennbridge, & Swofford, 1991). Survival sex exacerbates the problems associated with risky sexual behavior. Researchers have shown that the number of teenagers engaging in survival sex has been increasing since the 1970s. Rotheram-Borus & Gwadz (1993) estimated that one million teenagers resort to survival sex to support themselves.

Gay Youth

Between 1.1% and 2.5% of adolescent males self-identify as gay or bisexual, yet this small group represents the majority of HIV-infected adolescents (CDC, 2000b; French, Story, Remafedi, Resnick, & Blum, 1996; Garofalo, Wolf, Kessel, Palfrey, & DuRant, 1998; Sussman & Duffy, 1996). In 1999, 46% of reported HIV infections among adolescent males aged 13–19 years and 51% of cases among men aged 20–24 years were attributed to male-to-male sexual contact (CDC, 2001). Data on the sexual behaviors of male gay and bisexual youth indicate that these youth typically initiate sex at early ages (around 12.5 years), and have numerous sexual partners (median of 8 by age 15; Rosario, Meyer-Bahlburg, Hunter, & Gwadz, 1999; Rotheram-Borus et al., 1994). Among young gay men, about 50% have a history of sexual abuse (Rotheram-Borus et al., 1994), especially among youth infected with HIV (Anaya, Swendeman, & Rotheram-Borus, 2001).

Incarcerated Youth

Incarcerated youth engage in risky sexual behaviors to a greater extent than the general population of adolescents; some of the risky behaviors researchers have linked incarcerated youth to are: 1) more sexual activity, 2) a greater number of sexual partners, 3) less consistent contraception use, and 4) an earlier age at first intercourse relative to students in high school (DiClemente et al., 1991; Shalwitz, 1991). The prevalence of sexually transmitted diseases (STDs) among incarcerated youth is high (Brady, Baker, &

Neinstein, 1988; Shalwitz, 1991). In one study, sentinel surveillance surveys collected in juvenile detention centers in San Francisco between 1990 and 1995 showed that prior STD history was reported by 10.4% of respondents (1992–1995 only). STD history increased significantly during the 3-year period to 12% of youth (Kim, McFarland, Kellogg, & Katz, 1999). Pregnancy is another condition prevalent with delinquent females (Breuner & Farrow, 1995; Shalwitz, 1991). It has been estimated that at least 24,000 pregnant adolescents are arrested each year, or 670 per day (Breuner & Farrow, 1995). Incarcerated youth are also at greater risk for HIV infection due to the high levels of injecting drug use, unprotected sex, survival sex, and STD rates in detention facilities (Morris, Baker, Valentine, & Pennisi, 1998; Sweeney, Lindegren, Buehler, Onorato, & Janssen, 1995). Prevalence rates for inmate populations have been documented to be as high as 17.4% (Vlahov et al., 1991; Weisfuse et al., 1991). Vlahov et al. reported that 5.2% of women and 2.3% of men under 25 years of age were seropositive for HIV upon entrance into 10 selected correctional systems in moderate-to high-HIV prevalence areas within the east, west, and Midwest regions of the United States.

Psychiatrically Disturbed Youth

Several studies have examined risk behaviors among adolescents with psychiatric disorders. DiClemente et al. (1989) found that among a hospitalized sample of youth (N = 44), many risk behaviors were prevalent: intravenous drug use (15%), sharing of needles (15%), being a partner of an IV drug user (15.8%), being a sexual partner of a homosexual/bisexual male (15.8%), and having sex with someone whose sexual history is unknown (35%). In a related study, researchers found high levels of drug abuse (17% reported daily use of drugs), high-risk sexual activities (57%), and histories of STDs (17%) among a small sample of hospitalized girls (Baker & Mossman, 1991). Also, as previously mentioned, psychiatrically disturbed youth initiate sex at a very early age (mean of 10.7 years; DiClemente et al., 1989).

Urban Youth

Urban youth who live in high-poverty neighborhoods are at increased risk for negative developmental and health outcomes (Wilson, 1987). One such outcome is early sexual initiation (DiClemente et al., 1992; Keller et al., 1991), which in turn has been linked to (among other things) increased STD rates. As Hein (1989) has noted, geography is destiny; STD rates have been shown to be elevated among inner-city populations (Hatcher et al., 1986; Pratt et al., 1984). In one study, a clinic sample found that 16.8% of youth had STDs (Keller et al., 1991). Inner-city adolescent crack users in particular are at greater risk for STDs. One report showed that 41% of their sample had an STD, and significantly more girls (55%) than boys (34%) were affected (Fullilove, Fullilove, Bowser, & Gross, 1990). High pregnancy rates have also been linked to inner-city residency (Hayes, 1987; Hofferth & Hayes, 1987). Anderson (1989) argues that males living in inner cities have "sex codes" that value fathering a child as a sign of virility and status, which compensates for lack of job opportunities that normally would validate their manhood.

Factors Influencing Sexual Risk

Sexual risk acts among adolescents appear influenced by a variety of causes. Among these are: personality factors, family and peer influence, parental adjustment, personal religious beliefs, intelligence and educational aspirations, and parental communication and monitoring.

Personality Factors

Researchers have found that sexual risk behavior is influenced by one's psychological state. For example, the psychological construct of behavioral dysregulation is hypothesized as an underlying mechanism for antisocial behavior and substance abuse (Moffitt, 1993), as well as risky sexual behavior (Miller & Brown, 1991). Another construct—*behavioral dysregulation*—is defined as "an inability to inhibit maladaptive behaviors, thus prohibiting the effective execution of goal-directed plans" (Mezzich et al., 1997). It is characterized by "hyperactivity, impulsivity, inattention and aggression" (Martin et al., 1994). The personality trait of *negative affectivity* is also related to risky sexual behavior (Nyamathi, 1991; O'Leary, 1994). Negative affectivity includes aversive stress reactions, feelings of alienation, lack of emotional control, anxiety, and dysphoria (Mezzich et al., 1987; Watson & Clark, 1992). Helping adolescents develop behavioral routines to inhibit impulsive behaviors may be one effective strategy to reduce sexual risk that is not often implemented by intervention programs.

Intelligence and Educational Aspirations

A number of studies show a strong correlation between low intellectual ability, low achievement, lack of educational goals, and early sexual initiation among both African Americans and Caucasians. Adolescent girls who score low on intelligence tests and who also place little value on educational achievement are more likely to have intercourse at early ages than those who are educationally ambitious. Alternatively, research has shown that young girls who score higher on intelligence tests, are doing well in school, and are motivated to excel academically are less likely to engage in sex at a young age (Hogan & Kitagawa, 1983; Jessor, Costa, Jessor, & Donovan, 1983; Mott, 1983). Young men aged 17–20 showed similar results (Mott, 1983).

Personal Religious Beliefs

An individual's social group has been shown to impact behavior because of the group's influence on one's social identity (Bock, Beeghley, & Mixon, 1983; Cochran & Beeghley, 1991). One important social group is one's religious community (Bock et al., 1983). Many adolescents may not engage in sexually risky behaviors due both to their religious beliefs and the proscriptions of their particular faith (Cochran & Beeghley, 1991; Jessor, 1992; Woodroof, 1985). Alternatively, decreases in both church attendance and identification with religious group norms are associated with an increased probability of drinking and engaging in sexual activity among college students (Cochran & Beeghley, 1991; Reed & Meyers, 1991). Social group identification is an important component to examine when discussing individual behaviors.

Neighborhood and Peer Influence

Teenage sexual activity seems to be influenced by socioeconomic status. Teenagers from neighborhoods with higher socioeconomic status (as measured by neighborhood income, unemployment rate, or percent of households on welfare) have lower proportions of youth engaging in sexual intercourse. Teens with better educated mothers, and teens from two-parent families were also less likely to have had sexual intercourse (CDC, 2000b). Additionally, the *peer influence model* is based on the premise that peers greatly influence one another's behaviors (Catania, Kegeles, Coates, 1990; Jessor, Van Den Bos, Vanderryn, Costa, & Turbin, 1995). This model has been successfully used to increase knowledge about HIV infection as well as to reduce high-risk sexual behaviors among adolescents (Slap, Plotkin, Khalid, Michelman, & Forke, 1991).

Parental Influences

ADJUSTMENT. Many studies have linked dysfunctional family characteristics (e.g., parental alcohol abuse) to the social adjustment problems of children (Chandy, Harris, Blum, & Resnick, 1994); however, sexual behavior patterns are not typically linked to parents' behaviors. Rydelius (1981) finds that teenage girls from alcoholic families had more children than those who were not from alcoholic families. Female adult children of alcoholics report significantly higher rates of sexual dysfunction than others (Currier & Aponte, 1991), are more likely to be sexually active, and are more likely to become pregnant (Chandy et al., 1994). Childhood victimization (e.g., physical and sexual abuse) has consistently been associated with increased sexual risk, especially among young women (Chandy et al., 1994; Rotheram-Borus et al., 1996). In one study, researchers found that two-thirds of pregnant adolescent girls had been sexually abused and were less likely than their non-abused counterparts to use contraceptive measures consistently (Boyer & Fine, 1992). These studies underscore the influence that family characteristics can have on children's sexual behaviors.

COMMUNICATION. Parents and youth generally agree that being violent, using drugs, smoking cigarettes, or dropping out of school are negative events; however, parent and youth attitudes towards the age and context under which adolescents are to become sexually active are not consistent. Many adults believe that adolescents should delay sexual intercourse until marriage (Welbourne-Moglia & Edwards, 1986); however, adult expectations often do not match adolescents' pattern of sex behaviors (Romer et al., 1999). Consequently, policy decisions concerning adolescent sexuality are often made based on attitudes and desires, not research data (National Institutes of Mental Health [NIMH], 1997). Conversations about sexual behavior with adolescent children often generate anxiety in the parents; this anxiety inhibits the assistance parents can provide to help their children successfully achieve normal developmental milestones (Geasler, Dannison, & Edlund, 1995; Postrado & Nicholson, 1992). The parent's feelings are mirrored in the adolescents' feelings of personal inadequacy or awkwardness and reluctance or embarrassment in approaching their parents with the topic (Goldman & Goldman, 1981). The importance of parent-child communication cannot be underestimated. Parental communication about sexual risk acts was shown to increase the likelihood that adolescents used condoms in the past, and would continue to do so in the future (Romer et al., 1999). Early and clear communications between parents and young people is an important step in helping adolescents adopt and maintain protective sexual behaviors (CDC, 1999e).

MONITORING. Consistent parental monitoring (e.g., parents knowing where adolescents are after school, parents setting curfews, etc.) is a strategy associated with lower levels of adolescent risk behavior (Rodgers, 1999). Conversely, poor parental monitoring is associated with adolescent involvement in drug, alcohol, and tobacco use, jail, as well as sexual activity (e.g., Biglan et al., 1990; Fletcher, Darling, & Steinberg, 1994). Increasing parental monitoring is an intervention strategy currently being explored to reduce sexual risk acts (see Pequegnat & Szapocznik, 2000 for a review).

Effective Intervention Approaches

Programs to reduce adolescents' sexual risk are typically framed as adolescent AIDS prevention programs, pregnancy prevention, or programs to prevent sexually transmitted diseases. Effective programs for each of these categories have been repeatedly reviewed (e.g., Alan Guttmacher Institute, 1994; CDC, 2000a; Jemmott & Jemmott, 2000). Eight major approaches to reducing adolescents' risky sexual behaviors have been identified: 1) school-based programs; 2) school-based and school-linked clinics; 3) programs in community-based agencies; 4) parenting programs; 5) programs in health, mental health, and substance abuse treatment facilities; 6) peer-based programs; 7) community-level interventions; and 8) structural and policy interventions.

School-Based Interventions

Nationally, more than 90% of students receive education about AIDS or HIV infection in school (although Hispanic students reported significantly lower rates of receiving AIDS education; CDC, 2000e). The most effective school-based programs are comprehensive and focus on delaying the initiation of sexual behaviors and providing information on safe sex for those who are sexually active (CDC, 1999e). Because the school setting offers a logical and convenient way to reach youth, school-based interventions should continue to play an integral part in efforts to mitigate risky behaviors among adolescents. Two programs are recognized as successful: Reducing the Risks (Kirby, 2000) and Get Real About AIDS (CDC, 1999d). Each of these achieve success through curricula at multiple grade levels, including parents in the programs, focusing on social skills necessary to implement responsible sexual behavior, and providing access to resources (such as condoms).

Effective school-based programs share similar characteristics: (a) a narrow focus on reducing sexual risk behaviors; (b) being based on social learning theory; (c) including basic, accurate information about the risks of unprotected intercourse combined with experiential activities that personalize this information; (d) reinforcing specific, clear, and appropriate values to strengthen individual values and group norms against unprotected sex; (e) including activities that address social or media influences on sexual behaviors; (f) modeling and practice of skills; (g) using teaching methods that encourage student participation; (h) tailoring behavioral goals, material, and teaching methods to the age, experience, and culture of the students; (i) allowing sufficient time to complete important activities adequately; and (j) using trained teachers or peers who believed in the program (Kirby, 1999).

School-based programs come in two genres: Abstinence-only and abstinence-based prevention programs. Abstinence-only programs teach abstinence outside of marriage as the only viable option, with any discussion of contraception either forbidden or drastically limited (Institute of Medicine, 2000). Abstinence-based programs encourage abstinence, but include information and skills regarding methods of reducing sexual risk (Institute of Medicine, 2000). No research to date has shown that abstinence-only programs are effective (Jemmott & Jemmott, 2000; Kirby, 2000). Yet, the same day that a blue ribbon group of scientists indicated that abstinence-only programs are ineffective (NIMH, 1997), the federal government set aside $50 million to promote such programs. Such congressional action demonstrates the gap between scientifically based directions for policy and actual policy decision making (Institute of Medicine, 2000).

Many adolescents do not perceive sexual abstinence as an acceptable solution for AIDS prevention, and thus abstinence fails as an effective strategy (Hayes, 1987). One study found that at best, abstinence-based programs delay sexual intercourse for a maximum of 3 months (Jemmott, Jemmott, & Fong, 1998). However, several large school-based trials failed to demonstrate positive outcomes. For example, an AIDS education intervention for middle and high school aged youth in San Francisco improved students' knowledge of AIDS and reduced their fears of being infected by their HIV-positive classmates, but did not change their behavior (DiClemente et al., 1989).

Schools can be hostile environments for gay and lesbian youth (Savin-Williams, 1994), and most school districts in the United States do not offer prevention programs that address the needs of this seriously at-risk population (Rienzo, Button, & Wald, 1996). While gay youths are particularly vulnerable to such health-threatening problems as substance abuse, STDs, HIV/AIDS, homelessness, suicide, etc. (see for example, Savin-Williams, 1994; Unks, 1994), both researchers and students believe that schools hold great potential for reducing this vulnerability. Many problems exist with school-based programs targeted to gay, lesbian, and bisexual youth

(Rienzo et al., 1996). For one, school personnel often are not adequately prepared to address sexual orientation issues; they also often have a negative bias toward gay and lesbian youth (Tellijohann & Price, 1993; Kerr, Allensworth, & Gayle, 1989). For most homosexual youth, coming to terms with their sexual identity, as well as successfully navigating social and psychological development, is completed without assistance from the significant adults or institutions in their lives (Unks, 1994).

School-Based and School-Linked Clinics

As the problems of unintended pregnancy and STDs (most notably HIV/AIDS) have gained greater notoriety in society, about 40% of schools have sought to develop school-based and school-linked clinics to directly improve student access to contraceptives and STD treatment (Kirby, Waszak, & Ziegler, 1991). For a number of reasons, schools play an important role in reducing sexual risk-taking behaviors among adolescents. First, schools are the one institution in our society regularly attended by most people; approximately 95% of all youth five to 17 years old are enrolled in either elementary or secondary schools (National Center for Education Statistics, 1993). Second, virtually all youth attend school before the onset of sexual risk-taking behaviors and a majority is enrolled at the time of sexual initiation (Kirby, 2000). School-based clinics provide not only health care services for their students, but also an effective place through which to dispense contraceptives. As of Spring 2000, more than 1,300 centers are estimated to provide care in schools (Center for Health & Health Care in Schools, 2001). This is a substantial increase considering that, as of 1990, only 178 school-based clinics were operating (Hyche-Williams, 1990). The recent expansion has been fueled largely by state support; well over half of the 50 states promote the concept, either as a distinct initiative or as an option among a broader school-related health services program (Center for Health & Health Care in Schools, 2001).

Community-Based Programs

Community-based programs have the advantage of reaching youth who do not attend school, including homeless or runaway youth and school dropouts who live in difficult circumstances. Current approaches to HIV/AIDS interventions for such youth are based on the principal that education/intervention programs must address an individual's primary needs, and that these programs are best implemented by peers and trustworthy adults (Walters, 1999). A number of successful HIV-specific prevention programs have been identified. These randomized studies have demonstrated positive reductions in HIV risk acts (see Rotheram-Borus et al., 2000 for a review).

Almost all of these successful community-based interventions adopt the same format: small group, multiple session, and skills-focused cognitive behavioral programs. Street Smart is one example (Rotheram-Borus, Koopman, Haignere, & Davies, 1991; Rotheram-Borus et al., 2001). This program sought to reduce HIV risk behavior and increase condom use among runaways in New York City. Meeting over 10 sessions, youth were provided free condoms and comprehensive health care as the backdrop for the intervention. Within the group meetings, youth acquired the skills to negotiate safer sexual and substance use behaviors.

One study (Metzler, Biglan, Noell, Ary, & Ochs, 2000) has shown that an alternative intervention approach can also be successful in lessening sexual risk behaviors. This study differed from previous work on adolescent sexual risk reduction in two significant ways: 1) it examined the effectiveness of a behavior change intervention with adolescent STD clinic patients, and 2) the intervention utilized an individualized, rather than group approach common to studies on adolescents. Measured at six-month follow-up, participants had fewer sexual partners, fewer non-monogamous partners, and fewer sexual contacts with strangers in the past three months, when compared to a control group.

Most programs for lesbian and gay youth are provided by community-based agencies. Sexual activity between males is the primary mode of HIV infection for one third of adolescent males, and two thirds of the 20–24-year-old males (CDC, 2001). Like many other youth, young gay and bisexual men often do not consider their peers to be at risk for infection, and often do not have social support networks that encourage the practice of safer sex (CDC, 2001). Kegeles, Hays and Coates (1996) designed a community-level HIV prevention program for young gay men in a mid-sized Oregon community. The program was peer led and had 3 components: 1) outreach, 2) small groups, and 3) a publicity campaign. Independent from the prevention program, a cohort of 300 young gay men was surveyed both pre- and post-intervention, in this and a similar matched community. Following the intervention, the proportion of men engaging in any unprotected anal intercourse decreased from 20.2 to 11.1% (−45% from baseline) with non-primary partners, and from 58.9 to 44.7% (−24% from baseline) with boyfriends. No significant changes occurred in the comparison community over the same period. These researchers argued that their findings suggest that, to reach risk-taking young gay men, HIV prevention activities must be embedded in social activities and community life (Kegeles et al., 1996).

Parenting Programs

Although peers are traditionally seen as a source of normative influence, parents of adolescents are another potentially important and historically underutilized normative influence. Parents, particularly mothers, are key socializing agents in the lives of female adolescents (Rotheram-Borus, Murphy, & Miller, 1995), and interventions using them often aim to improve parental-adolescent communication. Parsons, Butler, Kocik, Norman, and Nuss (1998) examined the relationship between family communication and HIV risk reduction behaviors in a multi-site sample of 125 male youths (ages 12–25 years) with hemophilia and HIV infection, and their parents. Youth completed self-report surveys assessing communication and attitudes regarding HIV risk reduction. Adolescents also provided data about their sexual behaviors. Results indicated that adolescents who discuss sexual issues with parents are more likely to disclose their HIV status to sexual partners. Timing is an important factor to consider as well. The importance of reaching adolescents early was discussed by Rossi (1997), who recommended that youth be involved in sexual risk prevention programs between the ages of 8 and 14 (preferably as close to 8 as possible) in order to maximize the opportunity to reach early adolescents when they are most susceptible to parental influence.

There are several parental intervention programs in progress (see Pequegnat & Szapocznik, 2000 for a review). Given the longitudinal nature of these studies, the results will not be available for some time. The focus of these studies indicates that researchers are beginning to realize the importance of using the powerful influence that parents have on their children to reduce sexual risk behaviors of youth.

Prevention in Health, Mental Health, and Substance Abuse Treatment Settings

Most physicians do not discuss sexuality or sexual risk with their adolescent patients (Schuster, Bell, Petersen, & Kanouse, 1996), but when they do, there is a substantial reduction in risk behaviors (Fisher & Fisher, 1992). In addition, when persons are repeatedly interviewed about sexual risk, the number of sexual risk acts decreases (e.g., National Multi-Site of HIV Prevention, 1998). Some counties have implemented screening questionnaires in waiting rooms (e.g., Ventura county) and interventions are currently evaluating the strategy of repeated assessments in waiting rooms (e.g., Lightfoot, 2002). While the results of these studies are not conclusive, many observations suggest that inquiries regarding risk may result in risk reductions.

Parallel to the results from studies in community-based settings, successful interventions for adolescents in treatment settings (e.g., St. Lawrence, Jefferson, Alleyne, & Brasfield, 1995) are also based on small group, multiple-session, and skills-focused cognitive behavioral approaches. Youth in substance abuse treatment programs have high rates of sexual risk acts, as well as high rates of substance use, and drug prevention programs often address only needle sharing and substance use among these youth. Similarly, mental health researchers address only mental health problems; but sexual risk acts place both subpopulations at risk for negative outcomes other than sexual risk. While theories point to interrelationships between risk acts, the programs rarely are successful in more than one area of behavior. This challenges future prevention researchers to design effective programs that can be implemented in everyday settings and address multiple problem behaviors.

Peer-Based Programs

Peer relationships and the perceptions of peers can significantly impact a youth's protective behavior and should be a central focus of prevention programs (Stanton, Li, Galbraith, Feigelman, & Kaljee 1996). Peer groups can provide social arenas where sexual experimentation and initiation are encouraged. These young people also provide each other with special phrases, words, and sophisticated sexual vocabularies that they use to pursue, enact, and understand their sexual conduct (UNAIDS, 1999). Peer-based programs are an effective way to promote safe sex messages. In one study (Dunn, Ross, Caines, & Howorth, 1998), researchers evaluated a brief, randomly assigned, school-based HIV/AIDS prevention intervention for 9th graders delivered by either community health nurses (CHN) or by trained peer educators (PE). Based on post intervention survey responses, students in the PE-led group had significantly higher HIV knowledge scores than students in the CHN-led group. In addition, the PE-led group had significantly higher scores on HIV/AIDS prevention attitudes, self-efficacy, and behavioral intentions questionnaires than did a control group. On specific questionnaire items associated with condom use, scores indicated that the PE-led intervention, and to a lesser extent the CHN-led intervention, had a significant positive impact.

Community-Level Interventions

In the United States, two community-level interventions have been conducted, both in public housing facilities (Sikkema et al., 2000; Stanton et al., 1994). In both interventions, community activities and access to condoms and resources for health care were offered on an ongoing basis, in addition to small group, skill-focused meetings with teens. Movement in and out of the housing projects hampered evaluation of the long-term effects of the program. Yet, for broad dissemination of HIV prevention education, these are important opportunities and strategies that must be encouraged in the future to promote responsible sexuality and reductions in sexual risk behaviors.

Structural and Policy Interventions

Structural and policy-level interventions have the possibility of being broadly implemented in a relatively short time frame. For example, in addition to focusing on reducing unprotected sexual risk by programs targeting individuals, HIV prevention programs may reduce risk by expanding programs focused on such issues as economic development, social skills training, access to HIV testing, improved health care, and greater employment possibilities (Rotheram-Borus, 2000). Consequently, structural approaches to reducing sexual risk could include: funding and economic development programs, mandating delivery of HIV prevention programs at key developmental milestones (e.g., childbirth or marriage), and providing access to health care by increasing substantially the number of school-based and school-linked clinics, securing changes in legislative and funding policies through ballot initiatives or lawsuits, and privatizing prevention activities (Rotheram-Borus, 2000). To implement structural interventions for adolescents, however, requires that researchers shift their own armamentarium of strategies to include those used by lawyers, private enterprise, and lobbyists.

Summary

It is significant that both individual and social costs result from adolescents engaging in risky sexual behaviors. Much effort should be focused on helping young people achieve sexual responsibility. Such efforts require a comprehensive approach to understanding how adolescent behaviors vary by age, gender, racial/ethnic, and socioeconomic groups; how they evolve during the process of adolescent development; the disparate meanings and values within distinct adolescent cultures; and how family functioning and childhood experiences shape these behaviors and values.

An underlying theme permeating researchers' discussions about adolescent sexual risk behavior suggests that many of these behaviors can be tied to processes best explained within the context of *social identity theory*.

Social identity theory's premise centers on the presumption that an individual's behavior occurs in social situations and is influenced by various external factors exerting a substantial degree of influence on the behavior of the individual. Because individuals define themselves in terms of their group memberships, this social, self-defining perception therefore produces and shapes the social behavior and actions of individuals (Leyens, Yzerbyt, & Schadron, 1994). Such *social comparison* posits that individuals assess their own opinions and skills in comparison to others and these assessments, in turn, will have influence on the their behaviors.

The *peer-influence model* naturally extends social comparison and is based on the observation that adolescents are greatly influenced by their peers' behaviors (Jessor et al., 1995). The interventions based on the peer-influence model have prevented smoking, reduced alcohol use, increased knowledge about HIV infection, and most importantly, reduced high-risk sex and drug use behaviors (Booth et al., 1999; Slap et al., 1991). Adolescence is a time of experimentation and increased self-awareness when youth strive to develop their own identities (Jemmott & Jemmott, 1996). During this developmental period, adolescents also begin to experiment with different mating behaviors, and with risky behaviors such as drug and alcohol use, sex with multiple partners, etc., this can be best understood within the framework of social identity theory.

While this broader approach will help us better understand adolescent risk-taking, it is also true that although several researchers have designed and implemented effective sexual risk reduction programs, many of these programs have not yet been broadly disseminated. Public attitudes toward adolescents must change and policies must be recast to support evidence-based programs and to achieve broad dissemination. For example, potential interventions could be provided in workplaces, shopping malls, and faith communities, and theoretical models other than social cognitive models must be used. Given both the individual and social consequences of engaging in high-risk sexual behaviors, adolescents deserve nothing less.

References

Alan Guttmacher Institute. (1994). *Sex and America's teenagers*. New York: Author.

Anaya, H.D., Swendeman, D., & Rotheram-Borus, M.J. (2001). *Differences among abused and non-abused youth living with HIV/AIDS*. Manuscript submitted for publication.

Anderson, E. (1989). Sex codes and family life among poor inner-city youths. *Annals of the American Academy of Political and Social Sciences, 501*, 59–78.

Anderson, N.L.R., Koniak-Griffin, D., & Keenan, C.K. (1999). Evaluating the outcomes of parent-child family life education. *Scholarly Inquiry for Nursing Practice, 13*, 211–31.

Baker, D.G., & Mossman, D. (1991). Potential HIV exposure in psychiatrically hospitalized adolescent girls. *American Journal of Psychiatry, 148*, 528–30.

Berry, E.H., Shillington, A.M., Peak, T., & Hohman, M.M. (2000). Multi-ethnic comparison of risk and protective factors for adolescent pregnancy. *Child & Adolescent Social Work Journal, 17*, 79–96.

Biglan, A., Metzler, C.W., Wirt, R., Ary, D., Noell, J., Ochs, L., et al. (1990). Social and behavior factors associated with high-risk sexual behavior among adolescents. *Journal of Behavioral Medicine, 13*, 245–61.

Bock, E.W., Beeghley, L., & Mixon, A.J. (1983). Religion, socioeconomic status, and sexual morality: An application of reference group theory. *The Sociological Quarterly, 24*, 545–59.

Booth, R.E., Zhang, Y., & Kwiatkowski, C.F. (1999). The challenge of changing drug and sex risk behaviors of runaway and homeless adolescents. *Child Abuse & Neglect, 23*, 1295–1306.

Boyer, D., & Fine, D. (1992). Sexual abuse as a factor in adolescent pregnancy and child maltreatment. *Family Planning Perspectives, 24*, 4–11.

Brady, M., Baker, C., & Neinstein, L.S. (1988). Asymptomatic chlamydia trachomatis infections in teenage males. *Journal of Adolescent Health Care, 9*, 72–75.

Braverman, P.K., & Strasburger, V.C. (1994). Sexually transmitted diseases. *Clinical Pediatrics, 33*, 26–37.

Breakwell, G.M., Millward, L.J., & Fife-Schaw, C. (1994). Commitment to safer sex as a predictor of condom use among 16–20 year-olds. *Journal of Applied Social Psychology, 24*, 189–217.

Breuner, C.C., & Farrow, J.A. (1995). Pregnant teens in prison: Prevalence, management, and consequences. *Western Journal of Medicine, 162*, 328–30.

Catania, J.A., Kegeles, S.M., & Coates, T.J. (1990). Towards an understanding of risk behavior: An AIDS risk reduction model (ARRM). *Health Education Quarterly, 17*, 53–72.

Cates, W., Jr. (1990). The epidemiology of sexually transmitted diseases in adolescence. In M. Schydlower & M.A. Shafer (Eds.), *Adolescent medicine: State of the art reviews: AIDS and other sexually transmitted diseases* (pp. 409–27). Philadelphia: Hanley & Belfus.

Centers for Disease Control & Prevention. (1991). Premarital sexual experience among adolescent women—United States, 1970–1988. *Morbidity & Mortality Weekly Reports, 39*, 929–32.

Centers for Disease Control & Prevention. (1994). Health risk behaviors among adolescents who do and do not attend school—United States, 1992. *Morbidity & Mortality Weekly Report, 43*, 129–32.

Centers for Disease Control & Prevention. (1998a). Diagnosis and reporting of HIV and AIDS in states with integrated HIV and AIDS surveillance—United States, January 1994–June 1997. *Morbidity & Mortality Weekly Reports, 47*, 309–14.

Centers for Disease Control & Prevention. (1998b). Trends in sexual risk behaviors among high school students, United States, 1991–1997. *Morbidity & Mortality Weekly Reports, 47*, 749–52.

Centers for Disease Control & Prevention. (1999a). CDC Update: Status of perinatal HIV infection. Retrieved October 18, 2001 from: *http://www.hivpositive.com/f-Women/-VerticalTrans/CDC-updates/Vertical-HIV/perinatl.htm.*

Centers for Disease Control & Prevention. (1999b). Fact sheet: Sexual behavior. Retrieved October 18, 2001 from: *http://www.cdc.gov/nccdphp/dash/sexualbehaviorsfactsheet.htm.*

Centers for Disease Control & Prevention. (1999c). Fact sheet: Youth risk behavior trends. Retrieved October 18, 2001 from: *http://www.cdc.gov/nccdphp/dash/yrbs/trend.htm.*

Centers for Disease Control & Prevention. (1999d). Teen pregnancy. Retrieved October 18, 2001 from: *http://www.cdc.gov/nccdphp/teen.htm.*

Centers for Disease Control & Prevention. (1999e). *Young people at risk: HIV/AIDS among America's youth.* Retrieved October 18, 2001 from: *http://www.cdc.gov/hiv/pubs/facts/youth.htm.*

Centers for Disease Control and Prevention. (1999f). *Youth Risk Behavior Survey 1999.* Atlanta, GA: Author.

Centers for Disease Control & Prevention. (1999g). 1998 Sexually transmitted disease surveillance. Retrieved October 18, 2001 from: *http://www.cdc.gov/nchstp/dstd/Stats_Trends/1998_Surv_Rpt_main_pg.htm.*

Centers for Disease Control & Prevention. (2000a). Adolescent and school health: Programs that work. Retrieved October 18, 2001 from: *http://www.cdc.gov/nccdphp/dash/rtc/hiv-curric.htm.*

Centers for Disease Control & Prevention/National Center for Health Statistics. (2000b). *Health, United States, 2000 with adolescent health chartbook.* Retrieved October 18, 2001 from: *http://www.cdc.gov/nchs/data/hus00.pdf.*

Centers for Disease Control & Prevention/National Center for Health Statistics. (2000c). Trends in pregnancies and pregnancy rates by outcome: Estimates for the United States. *Vital & Health Statistics, 21*(56).

Centers for Disease Control & Prevention. (2000d). Variations in teenage birth rates, 1991–98: National and state trends. *National Vital Statistics Reports, 48*(6).

Centers for Disease Control & Prevention. (2000e). Youth risk behavior surveillance—United States, 1999. *Morbidity & Mortality Weekly Reports, 49*, No. SS-5, 1–104.

Centers for Disease Control & Prevention. (2001). *Fact sheet: Need for sustained HIV prevention among men who have sex with men.* Retrieved October 18, 2001 from: *http://www.cdc.gov/hiv/pubs/facts/msm.htm.*

The Center for Health & Health Care in Schools. (2001). *1999–2000 Survey of school-based health center initiatives: Number of centers and state financing.* Retrieved October 18, 2001 from: *http://www.healthinschools.org/sbhcs/sbhcs_table.htm.*

Chandy, J.M., Harris, L., Blum, R.W., & Resnick, M.D. (1994). Female daughters of alcohol misusers: Sexual behaviors. *Journal of Youth and Adolescence, 23*, 695–709.

Cleland, J., & Ferry, B. (Eds.). (1995). *Sexual behaviour and AIDS in the developing world.* London: Taylor & Francis.

Cochran, J.K., & Beeghley, L. (1991). The influence of religion on attitudes toward nonmarital sexuality: A preliminary assessment of reference group theory. *Journal for the Study of Religion, 30*, 45–62.

Crowe, L.C., & George, W.H. (1989). Alcohol and human sexuality: Review and integration. *Psychological Bulletin 105*, 374–386.

Currier, K.D., & Aponte, J.F. (1991). Sexual dysfunction in female adult children of alcoholics. *International Journal of the Addictions, 26*, 195–201.

DiClemente, R.J., Durbin, M., Siegel, D., Krasnovsky, F., Lazarus, N., & Comacho, T. (1992). Determinants of condom use among junior high school students in a minority, inner-city school district. *Pediatrics, 89*, 197.

DiClemente, R.J., Lanier, M.M., Horan, P.F., & Lodico, M. (1991). Comparison of AIDS knowledge, attitudes, and behaviors among incarcerated adolescents and a public school sample in San Francisco. *American Journal of Public Health, 81*, 628–30.

DiClemente, R.J., Ponton, L.E., Hartley, D., & McKenna, S. (1989). Prevalence of HIV-related high-risk sexual and drug-related behaviors among psychiatrically hospitalized adolescents: Preliminary results. In J. Woodrull, D. Doherty & A.J. Garrison (Eds.), *Troubled adolescents and HIV infection: Issues in prevention and treatment* (pp. 70–88). Washington, DC: Georgetown University.

Donovan, J.E., Jessor, R., & Costa, F.M. (1991). Adolescent health behavior and conventiona-lity-unconventionality: An extension of problem-behavior theory. *Health Psychology, 10,* 53–61.

Dunn, L., Ross, B., Caines, T., & Howorth, P. (1998). A school-based HIV/AIDS prevention edu-cation program: Outcomes of peer-led versus community health nurse-led interventions. *Canadian Journal of Human Sexuality, 7,* 339–45.

Elliott, D.S., & Morse, B.J. (1989). Delinquency and drug use as risk factors in teenage sexual activity. *Youth and Society, 21,* 32–60.

Fisher, J.D., & Fisher, W.A. (1992). Changing AIDS-risk behavior. *Psychological Bulletin, 111,* 455–74.

Fletcher, A.C., Darling, N., & Steinberg, L. (1994). Parental monitoring and peer influences on adolescent substance use. In J. McCord (Ed.), *Coercion and punishment in long-term perspectives* (pp. 259–71). New York: Cambridge University Press.

French, S.A., Story, M., Remafedi, G., Resnick, M.D., & Blum, R.W. (1996). Sexual ori-entation and prevalence of body dissatisfaction and eating disordered behaviors: A population-based study of adolescents. *International Journal of Eating Disorders, 19,* 119–26.

Fullilove, R.E., Fullilove, M.T., Bowser, B.P., & Gross, S.A. (1990). Risk of sexually transmitted disease among black adolescent crack users in Oakland and San Francisco, California. *Journal of the American Medical Association, 263,* 851.

Garofalo, R., Wolf, R.C., Kessel, S., Palfrey, J., & DuRant, R.H. (1998). The association between health risk behaviors and sexual orientation among a school-based sample of adolescents. *Pediatrics, 101,* 895–902.

Geasler, M.J., Dannison, L.L., & Edlund, C.J. (1995). Sexuality education of young children: Parental concerns. *Family Relations, 44,* 184–88.

Gittes, E.B., & Irwin, C.E. (1993). Sexually transmitted diseases in adolescents. *Pediatrics in Review, 14,* 180–89.

Goldman, R.J., & Goldman, D.G. (1981). Sources of sex information for Australian, English, North American, and Swedish children. *Journal of Psychology, 109,* 87–92.

Hatcher, R.A., Guest, F., Stewart, F.H., Steart, G.K., Trussell, J., Cerel, S., et al. (1986). *Contraceptive technology, 1986–1987.* New York: Irvington.

Hatcher, R.A., Trussell, J., Stewart, F., Stewart, G.K., Kowal, D., Guest, F., et al. (1994). *Contraceptive technology* (16th ed.). New York: Irvington.

Hayes, C.D. (1987). *Risking the future: Adolescent sexuality, pregnancy, and childbearing.* Washington, DC: National Academy Press.

Hein, K. (1989). AIDS in adolescence: Exploring the challenge. *Journal of Adolescent Health Care, 10,* 10S–35S.

Hein, K., Dell, R., Futterman, D., Rotheram-Borus, M.J., & Shaffer, N. (1995). Comparison of HIV+ and HIV− adolescents: Risk factors and psychosocial determinants. *Pediatrics, 95,* 96–104.

Henshaw, S.K. (1991). The accessibility of abortion services in the United States. *Family Plan-ning Perspectives, 23,* 246–52.

Hingson, R., Strunin, L., Berlin, B., & Heeren, T. (1990). Beliefs about AIDS, use of alcohol and drugs, and unprotected sex among Massachusetts adolescents. *American Journal of Public Health, 80,* 295–99.

Hofferth, S.L., & Hayes, C.D. (1987). *Risking the future: Adolescent sexuality, pregnancy, and childbearing, Volume 2.* Washington, D.C: National Academy Press.

Hofferth, S.L., & Moore, K.A. (1979). Early child bearing and later economic well-being. *American Sociological Review, 44,* 784–815.

Hogan, D.P., & Kitagawa, E.M. (1983, April). *Family factors in the fertility of Black adolescents.* Paper presented at the annual meeting of the Population Association of America, Pittsburgh, PA.

Hollander, D. (1996). Nonmarital childbearing in the United States: A government report. *Family Planning Perspectives, 28*, 29–32 & 41.

Hoyert. L., Kochanek, K.D., & Murphy, S.L. (1999). Deaths: Final data for 1997. *National Vital Statistics Reports, 47*, 1–104.

Hyche-Williams, H. (1990). *School-based clinics: Update 1990.* Washington, DC: The Center for Population Options, 12.

Institute of Medicine. (2000). *No time to lose: Getting more from HIV prevention.* Washington, DC: National Academy Press.

Jemmott, J.B. & Jemmott, L.S. (1993). Alcohol and drug use during sexual activity: Predicting the HIV-risk-relating behaviors of inner city Black male adolescents. *Journal of Adolescent Research, 8*, 41–57.

Jemmott, J.B. & Jemmott, L.S. (1996). Strategies to reduce the risk of HIV infection, sexually transmitted diseases, and pregnancy among African American adolescents. In R.J. Resnick & R.H. Rozensky (Eds.), *Health psychology through the life span: Practice and research opportunities.* (pp. 395–422). Washington, DC: American Psychological Assn.

Jemmott, J.B., & Jemmott, L.S. (2000). HIV behavioral interventions for adolescents in community settings. In J.L. Peterson & R.J. DiClemente (Eds.), *Handbook of HIV prevention.* (pp. 103–27). New York: Kluwer Academic/Plenum.

Jemmott, J.B., Jemmott, L.S., & Fong, G.T. (1998). Abstinence and safer sex HIV risk-reduction interventions for African American adolescents. *Journal of the American Medical Association, 279*, 1529–36.

Jessor, R. (1992). Risk behavior in adolescence: A psychological framework for understanding and action. *Developmental Review, 12*, 374–90.

Jessor, R., Costa, F., Jessor, S.L., & Donovan, J.E. (1983). The time of first intercourse: A prospective study. *Journal of Personality and Social Psychology, 44*, 608–26.

Jessor, S., & Jessor, R. (1977). *Problem behavior and psychological development: A longitudinal study of youth.* New York: Academic Press.

Jessor, R., Van Den Bos, J., Vanderryn, J., Costa, F.M., & Turbin, M.S. (1995). Protective factors in adolescent problem behavior: Moderator effects and developmental change. *Developmental Psychology, 31*, 923–33.

Keeling, R.P. (1988). *Beyond AIDS 101.* Paper presented at the AIDS Education Symposium, Boston, MA. April 1988.

Kegeles, S.M., Hays, R.B., & Coates, T.J. (1996). The Mpowerment Project: A community-level HIV prevention intervention for young gay men. *American Journal of Public Health, 86*, 1129–36.

Keller, S.E., Bartlett, J.A., Schleifer, S.J., Johnson, R.L., Pinner, E., & Delaney, B. (1991). HIV-relevant sexual behavior among a healthy inner-city heterosexual adolescent population in an endemic area of HIV. *Journal of Adolescent Health, 12*, 44–48.

Kerr, D.L., Allensworth, D.D., & Gayle, J.A. (1989). The ASHA national HIV education needs assessment of health and education professionals. *Journal of School Health, 59*, 301–07.

Kim, A.A., McFarland, W., Kellogg, T., & Katz, M.H. (1999). Sentinel surveillance for HIV infection and risk behavior among adolescents entering juvenile detention in San Francisco: 1990–1995.*AIDS, 13*, 1597–98.

Kirby, D. (1999). Sexuality and sex education at home and school. *Adolescent Medicine, 10*, 195–209.

Kirby, D. (2000). School-based interventions to prevent unprotected sex and HIV among adolescents. In J.L. Peterson & R.J. DiClemente (Eds.), *Handbook of HIV Prevention* (pp. 280–287). New York: Kluwer Academic/Plenum.

Kirby, D., Waszak, C., & Ziegler, J. (1991). Six school-based clinics: Their reproductive health services and impact on sexual behavior. *Family Planning Perspectives, 23*, 6–16.

Klanger, B., Tyden, T., & Ruusuvaara, L. (1993). Sexual behaviour among adolescents in Uppsala, Sweden. *Journal of Adolescent Health, 14*, 468–74.

Koniak-Griffin, D., & Brecht, M. (1995). Linkages between sexual risk taking, substance use, and AIDS knowledge among pregnant adolescents and young mothers. *Nursing Research, 44*, 340–46.

Ku, L., Sonenstein, F.L., & Pleck, J.H. (1993). Neighborhood, family, and work: Influences on the premarital behaviors of adolescent males. *Social Forces, 72*, 479–503.

Leyens, J.P., Yzerbyt, V., & Schadron, G. (1994). *Stereotypes and social cognition.* Thousand Oaks, CA: Sage.

Lightfoot, M. (2002). *Interventions for HIV positive adults in medical care settings.* Manuscript in preparation.

Martin, C.S., Earlywine, M., Blackson, T.C., Vanyukov, M.M., Moss, H.B., & Tarter, R.E. (1994). Aggressivity, inattention, hyperactivity, and impulsivity in boys at high and low risk for substance abuse. *Journal Abnormal Child Psychology, 22*, 177–203.

Maxwell, A., Bastani, R., & Yan, K. (1995). AIDS risk behaviors and correlates in teenagers attending sexually transmitted disease clinics in Los Angeles. *Genitourinary Medicine, 71*, 82–87.

McQuillan, G.M., Khare, M., Kareon, J.M., Schable, C.A., & Vlahov, D. (1997). Update on the seroepidemiology of human immunodeficiency virus in the United States household population: NHANES III, 1988–1994. *Journal of Acquired Immune Deficiency Syndromes and Human Retrovirology, 14*, 355–60.

Melchert, T., & Burnett, K.F. (1990). Attitudes, knowledge, and sexual behavior of high-risk adolescents: Implications for counseling and sexuality education. *Journal of Counseling & Development, 68*, 293–98.

Metzler, C.W., Biglan, A., Noell, J., Ary, D.V., & Ochs, L. (2000). A randomized controlled trial of a behavioral intervention to reduce high-risk sexual behavior among adolescents in STD clinics. *Behavior Therapy, 31*, 27–54.

Mezzich, A.C., Tarter, R.E., Giancola, P.R., Lu, S., Kirisci, L., & Parks, S. (1997). Substance use and risky sexual behavior in female adolescents. *Drug and Alcohol Dependence, 44*, 157–66.

Miller, W., & Brown, J. (1991). Self-regulation as a conceptual basis for the prevention of addictive behaviours. In N. Heather, W. Miller & J. Greeley (Eds.), *Self-control and the addictive behaviours* (pp. 3–79). Sydney, Australia: Maxwell Macmillian.

Moffitt, T.E. (1993). Adolescence-limited and life-course-persistent antisocial behavior: A developmental taxonomy. *Psychological Review, 100*, 674–701.

Moore, K.A., & Waite, L.J. (1981). Marital dissolution, early motherhood and early marriage. *Social Forces, 60*, 20–40.

Morris, R.E., Baker, C.J. Valentine, M., & Pennisi, A.J. (1998). Variations in HIV risk behaviors of incarcerated juveniles during a four-year period: 1989–1992. *Journal of Adolescent Health, 23*, 39–48.

Mott, F.L. (1983, November). *Early fertility behavior among American youth: Evidence from the 1982 national longitudinal surveys of labor force behavior of youth.* Paper presented at the annual meeting of the American Public Health Association, Dallas, TX.

Mott, F.L., & Haurin, R.J. (1988). Linkages between sexual activity and alcohol and drug use among American adolescents. *Family Planning Perspectives, 20*, 128.

National Center for Education Statistics. (1993). *Digest of Education Statistics.* Washington, DC: U.S. Department of Education.

National Center for Education Statistics. (1998). *Digest of education statistics, 1998.* Washington, DC: U.S. Department of Education.

National Center for Health Statistics, Centers for Disease Control and Prevention. (2000). Deaths: Final data for 1998. *National Vital Statistics Reports, 48,* 1–106.

National Institutes of Mental Health. (1997). *The National Institute of Mental Health Consensus Development Conference on Interventions to Prevent HIV Risk Behaviors: Program and Abstracts.* Bethesda, MD: NIMH.

National Institute of Mental Health Multisite HIV Prevention Trial Group. (1998). The NIMH Multisite HIV Prevention Trial: Reducing HIV sexual risk behavior. *Science, 280,* 1889–94.

Nyamathi, A. (1991). Relationship of resources to emotional distress, somatic complaints, and high-risk behaviors in drug recovery and homeless minority women. *Research in Nursing and Health, 14,* 269–77.

O'Leary, A. (1994). Factors associated with sexual risk of AIDS in women. *NIDA Research Monograph, 143:* 64–81.

Parsons, J.T., Butler, R., Kocik, S., Norman, L., & Nuss, R. (1998). The role of the family system in HIV risk reduction: Youths with hemophilia and HIV infection and their parents. *Journal of Pediatric Psychology, 23,* 57–65.

Pequegnat, W., & Szapocznik, J. (2000). *Working with families in the era of HIV/AIDS.* Thousand Oaks, CA: Sage.

Postrado, L., & Nicholson, H. (1992). Effectiveness in delaying initiation of sexual intercourse of girls aged 12–14: Two components of the Girls Incorporated Preventing Adolescent Pregnancy Program. *Youth and Society, 23,* 356–79.

Pratt, W., Mosher, W., Bachrach, C., & Horn, M. (1984). Understanding U.S. fertility: Findings from the National Survey of Family Growth, Cycle III. *Population Bulletin, 39,* 1–42.

Reed, L.A., & Meyers, L.S. (1991). A structural analysis of religious orientation and its relation to sexual attitudes. *Educational and Psychological Measurement, 51,* 943–52.

Remafedi, G. (1994). Cognitive and behavioral adaptations to HIV/AIDS among gay and bisexual adolescents. *Journal of Adolescent Health, 15,* 142–48.

Rienzo, B.A., Button, J., & Wald, K.D. (1996). The politics of school-based programs which address sexual orientation. *Journal of School Health, 66,* 33–40.

Robertson, M.J. (1989, April). *Homeless youth: An overview of recent literature.* Paper presented at the National Conference on Homeless Children and Youth, Washington, DC.

Rodgers, K.B. (1999). Parenting processes related to sexual risk-taking behaviors of adolescent males and females. *Journal of Marriage & the Family, 61,* 99–109.

Romer, D., Stanton, B., Galbraith, J., Feigelman, S., Black, M.M., & Li, X. (1999). Parental influence on adolescent sexual behavior in high-poverty settings. *Archives of Pediatric and Adolescent Medicine, 153,* 1055–62.

Rosario, M., Meyer-Bahlburg, H., Hunter, J., & Gwadz, M. (1999). Sexual risk behaviors of gay, lesbian, and bisexual youths in New York City: Prevalence and correlates. *AIDS Education & Prevention, 11,* 476–96.

Rosenbaum, E., & Kandel, D.B. (1990). Early onset of adolescent sexual behavior and drug involvement. *Journal of Marriage & the Family, 52,* 783–98.

Rossi, A.S. (1997). The impact of family structure and social change on adolescent sexual behavior. *Children and Youth Services Review, 19,* 369–400.

Rotheram-Borus, M.J. (2000). Expanding the range of interventions to reduce HIV among adolescents. *AIDS, 14*(Suppl. 1), S33–40.

Rotheram-Borus, M.J., & Gwadz, M. (1993). Sexuality among youths at high risk. *Psychiatric Clinics of North America, 2,* 415–30.

Rotheram-Borus, M.J., & Koopman, C. (1991). Safer sex and adolescence. In R.M. Lerner, A.C. Petersen, & J. Brooks-Gunn (Eds.), *Encyclopedia of adolescence* (pp. 951–60). New York: Garland.

Rotheram-Borus, M.J., Koopman, C., & Bradley, J. (1989). Barriers to successful AIDS prevention programs with runaway youth. In J.O. Woodruff, D. Doherty & J.G. Athey (Eds.), *Troubled adolescents and HIV infection: Issues in prevention and treatment* (pp. 37–55). Washington, DC: Janis.

Rotheram-Borus, M.J., Koopman, C., Haignere, C., & Davies, M. (1991). Reducing HIV sexual risk behaviors among runaway adolescents. *Journal of the American Medical Association, 266*, 1237–41.

Rotheram-Borus, M.J., Mahler, K.A., Koopman, C., & Langabeer, K. (1996). Sexual abuse history and associated multiple risk behavior in adolescent runaways. *American Journal of Orthopsychiatry, 66*, 390–400.

Rotheram-Borus, M.J., Meyer-Bahlburg, H., Rosario, M., Koopman, C., Haignere, C., Exner, T., et al. (1992). Lifetime sexual behaviors among predominantly minority male runaways and gay/bisexual adolescents in New York City. *AIDS Education and Prevention, Fall*(Suppl.), 34–42.

Rotheram-Borus, M.J., Murphy, D.A., Coleman, C.L., Kennedy, M., Reid, H.M., Cline, T.R., et al. (1997). Risk acts, health care, and medical adherence among HIV + youths in care over time. *AIDS and Behavior, 1*, 43–52.

Rotheram-Borus, M.J., Murphy, D.A., & Miller, S. (1995). Preventing AIDS in female adolescents. In A. O'Leary & L.S. Jemmott (Eds.), *Women at risk: Issues in the primary prevention of AIDS* (pp. 103–129). New York: Plenum.

Rotheram-Borus, M.J., O'Keefe, Z., Kracker, R., & Foo, H.-H. (2000). Prevention of HIV among adolescents. *Prevention Science, 1*, 15–30.

Rotheram-Borus, M.J., Rosario, M., Meyer-Bahlburg, H., Koopman, C., Dopkins, S., & Davies, M. (1994). Sexual and substance use acts among gay and bisexual male adolescents in New York City. *The Journal of Sex Research, 31*, 47–57.

Rotheram-Borus, M.J., Song, J., Gwadz, M., Lee, M., Van Rossem, R., & Koopman C. (2001). *Reductions in HIV risk among runaway youth.* Manuscript in preparation.

Rydelius, P.A. (1981). Children of alcoholic fathers: Their social adjustment and their health status over 20 years. *Acta Paediatrica Scandinavica Supplementum 286*, 1–89.

Savin-Williams, R.C. (1994). Verbal and physical abuse as stressors in the lives of lesbian, gay males, and bisexual youth: Associations with school problems, running away, substance abuse, prostitution and suicide. *Journal of Consulting & Clinical Psychology, 62*, 262–69.

Schwartz, I. (1993). Affective reactions of American and Swedish women to their first premarital coitus: A cross-cultural comparison. *Journal of Sex Research, 30*, 18–26.

Schuster, M.A., Bell, R.M., Petersen, L.P., & Kanouse, D.E. (1996). Communication between adolescents and physicians about sexual behavior and risk prevention. *Archives of Pediatrics and Adolescent Medicine, 150*, 906–13.

Shalwitz, J. (1991). The medical health status of incarcerated youth. In P.M. Sheahan (Ed.), *Health care of incarcerated youth: Report from the 1991 Tri-regional Workshops.* Washington, DC: National Center for Education in Maternal and Child Health.

Sikkema, K.J., Kelly, J.A., Winett, R.A., Solomon, L.J., Cargill, V.A., Roffman, R.A., et al. (2000). Outcomes of a randomized community-level HIV prevention intervention for women living in 18 low-income housing developments. *American Journal of Public Health, 90*, 57–63.

Singh S., & Darroch J.E. (2000). Adolescent pregnancy and childbearing: levels and trends in industrialized countries. *Family Planning Perspectives, 32*, 14–22.

Slap, G.B., Plotkin, M.S., Khalid, N., Michelman, D.F., & Forke, C.M. (1991). A human immunodeficiency virus peer education program for adolescent females. *Journal of Adolescent
Health, 12*, 434–42.

St. Lawrence, J.S., Jefferson, K.W., Alleyne, E., & Brasfield, T.L. (1995). Comparison of education versus behavioral skills training interventions in lowering sexual HIV-risk behavior of substance-dependent adolescents. *Journal of Consulting and Clinical Psychology, 63*,
154–57.

Stanton, B., Li, X., Black, M., Ricardo, I., Galbraith, J., Kaljee, L., et al. (1994). Sexual practices
and intentions among preadolescent and early adolescent low-income urban African-
Americans. *Pediatrics, 93*, 966–73.

Stanton, B.F., Li, X., Galbraith, J., Feigelman, S., & Kaljee, L. (1996). Sexually transmitted diseases, human immunodeficiency virus, and pregnancy prevention. Combined contraceptive practices among urban African-American early adolescents. *Archives of Pediatrics
and Adolescent Medicine, 150*, 17–24.

Stattin, H., & Magnusson, D. (1990). *Pubertal maturation in female development.* Hillsdale, NJ:
Earlbaum Associates.

Stiffman, A.R., Dore, P., Earls, F., & Cunningham, R. (1992). The influence of mental health
problems on AIDS-related risk behaviors in young adults. *The Journal of Nervous and
Mental Disease, 180*, 314–20.

Strunin, L., & Hingson, R. (1992). Alcohol, drugs, and adolescent sexual behavior. *International
Journal of the Addictions, 27*, 129–46.

Sussman, T., & Duffy, M. (1996). Are we forgetting about gay male adolescents in AIDS-related
research and prevention? *Youth & Society, 27*, 379–93.

Sweeney, P., Lindegren, M.L., Buehler, J.W., Onorato, I.M., & Janssen, R.S. (1995). Teenagers
at risk of human immunodeficiency virus type 1 infection. Results from seroprevalence surveys in the United States. *Archives of Pediatrics & Adolescent Medicine, 149*,
521–28.

Taylor, H., Kagay, M., & Leichenko, S. (1986). *American teens speak: Sex myths, TV, and birth
control.* New York: Planned Parenthood Federation of America.

Tellijohann, S.K., & Price, J.H. (1993). A qualitative examination of adolescent homosexuals'
life experiences: Ramifications for secondary school personnel. *Journal of Homosexuality,
26*(1), 41–56.

UNAIDS/WHO. (1998a). *AIDS epidemic update: December 1998.* Washington, DC: Author.

UNAIDS/WHO. (1998b). *Report on the global HIV/AIDS epidemic, June 1998.* Washington, DC:
Author.

UNAIDS/WHO. (1998c). *Statement for the World Conference of Ministers Responsible for Youth.*
Washington, DC: Author.

UNAIDS. (1999). *Sex and youth: Contextual factors affecting risk for HIV/AIDS. A comparative
analysis of multi-site studies in developing countries. Part One: Young people and risk-taking
in sexual relations.* Retrieved on October 11, 2001, from *http://www.unaids.org/publications/
documents/children/children/sexandyouth99.html*

Unks, G. (1994). Thinking about the homosexual adolescent. *The High School Journal, 77*, 1–6.

Vaglum, S., & Vaglum, P. (1987). Differences between alcoholic and non-alcoholic female
psychiatric patients. *Acta Psychiatrica Scandanavica, 76*, 309–16.

Ventura, S.J., Curtin, S.C., & Mathews, M.S. (2000). Variations in teenage birth rates, 1991–98:
National and state trends. *National Vital Statistics Reports, 48*(6).

Vlahov, D., Brewer, T.F., Castro, K.G., Narkunas, J.P., Salive, M.E., Ullrich, J., et al. (1991).
Prevalence of anti-body to HIV among entrants to U.S. correctional facilities. *Journal of
the American Medical Association, 265*, 1129–32.

Walters, A.S. (1999). HIV prevention in street youth. *Journal of Adolescent Health, 25*, 187–98.

Watson, D., & Clark, L.A. (1992). Affects separable and inseparable: On the hierarchical arrangement of negative affects. *Journal of Personality and Social Psychology, 62*, 489–505.

Weisfuse, I.B., Greenberg, B.L., Back, S.D., Makki, H.A., Thomas, P., Rooney, W.C., et al. (1991). HIV-1 infection among New York City inmates. *AIDS, 5*, 1133–38.

Welbourne-Moglia, A., & Edwards, S.R. (1986). Sex education must be stopped! *SIECUS Reports, 15*, 1–3.

Wellings, K., Wadsworth, J., Johnson, A., Field, J., Whitaker, L., & Field, B. (1995). Provision of sex education and early sexual experience: The relation examined. *British Medical Journal, 311*, 417–20.

Werdelin, L., Misfeldt, J., Melbye, M., & Olsen, J. (1995). An update on knowledge and sexual behaviour among students in Greenland. *Scandinavian Journal of Social Medicine, 20*, 158–64.

Wilson, W.J. (1987). *The truly disadvantaged.* Chicago, IL: University of Chicago Press.

Woodroof, James T. (1985). Religiosity and reference groups: Towards a model of adolescent sexuality (Doctoral dissertation, University of Nebraska, Lincoln, 1985). *Dissertation Abstracts International, 45*, 9-A, 3002–03.

Yates, G.L., Mackenzie, R.G., Pennbridge, J., & Swofford, A. (1991). A risk profile comparison of homeless youth involved in prostitution and homeless youth not involved. *Journal of Adolescent Health, 12*, 545–48.

Zelnik, M., & Shah, F. (1983). First intercourse among young Americans. *Family Planning Perspectives, 15*, 64–72

Zide, M.R., & Cherry, A.L. (1992). A typology of runaway youths: An empirically based definition. *Child & Adolescent Social Work Journal, 9*, 155–68.

Chapter 6

The Generic Features of Effective Childrearing

Anthony Biglan

Chapters 2 through 5 provide valuable summaries of the programs and policies that are available to prevent important problem behaviors. Each chapter is based on substantial empirical evidence from randomized controlled trials and interrupted time-series experimental evaluations. The widespread effective implementation of such well-evaluated practices is likely to contribute to substantial reductions in these problems in our society.

The present chapter takes a different, yet complementary, approach. It describes the generic features of environments that cultivate the successful development of children and adolescents. Each of the programs and policies described in previous chapters has one or more of these generic features. By identifying these features, we may be able to find other ways in which these practices can be fostered.

Programs and policies tend to have an impact in a limited domain. A school-based prevention program reaches young people in the school setting, but has limited impact on reducing family, neighborhood, or even peer influences on youth behavior. A policy targeting the reduction of youth access to alcohol affects the use of only one substance. Yet, the principles that are employed in these programs or policies might have an impact in other settings, if only they were applied. Identifying the generic features of childrearing might tell us how we can generalize effective practices to new settings. For example, many of the programs and practices involve the use of reinforcement to increase desirable behavior. Knowing the value of reinforcement in these programs should prompt us to find many other ways in which communities can increase reinforcement for desirable behavior.

Another reason for articulating generic principles is that communities are likely to continue to invent their own approaches to improving outcomes for kids, no matter how many blue ribbon panels identify and advocate for the adoption of empirically supported programs and policies. It is from these innovations that many of the improvements in outcomes for kids are likely to result. It would seem that the chances of these innovations making a difference would improve if they were guided by an understanding of the generic features of existing empirically supported programs.

Generic principles may also be generative. Knowledge of those principles may enable members of communities to modify existing practices or create new ones that enhance youth development in ways that have not been identified by existing research.

Generic principles are also relevant to the growing emphasis on positive youth development. Although empirical evidence remains exceedingly sparse, some have argued that it is important for communities not simply to focus on preventing problem behaviors, but to create an environment that nurtures the expansion of young people's skills and involvements. Generic principles could assist communities in attending to positive youth development in a way that solely implementing practices designed to prevent specific problems may not.

A final reason for identifying a set of generic child-rearing features is the fact that most adolescent problem behaviors are interrelated and influenced by the same environmental features. This suggests that we may be able to identify a small number of environmental features that prevent the development of diverse problems while enhancing diverse prosocial skills.

The empirical support for the importance of the features described here is substantial. However, it is of a different sort than the empirical evidence that supports the efficacy of specific programs and policies. In most cases, programs and policies have been evaluated in experimental evaluations (randomized trials or interrupted time-series experiments). The features described here are more like components of complex programs. In principle, it would be possible to tease out the effects of individual components of complex programs through randomized controlled trials that compare programs with and without a given component. Such studies are extremely costly and few of them have been done. However, the importance of these generic features comes not only from the fact that they are components of successful programs and policies, but also from considerable etiological research showing that these features of the environment are related to the development or prevention of numerous child and adolescent problem behaviors (e.g., Hawkins, Catalano, & Miller, 1992). Moreover, some of the components, such as reinforcement, have been shown in hundreds of experimental and correlations studies to be a critical influence on human behavior (Biglan, 1995).

A Focus on Communities

As a practical matter, many of the factors that influence childrearing out-comes are at the community level. School practices typically are set at the community level and certainly any policies that might be created would be set at the community level or at a higher level of political organization, such as the county or state. But even where the focus is on improving fam-ily management, community level factors are important. The systems that support and influence families, including schools, churches, and public and private family service agencies are often organized at the community level. And even where the coordination among these entities is weak or nonexistent at present, efforts to bring about better coordination among them are probably best organized at the community level.

There are also important scientific reasons for focusing on commu-nities as the chief unit of childrearing. The ultimate value of preventive efforts must be measured in terms of their ability to reduce the incidence and prevalence of problems in defined populations. Geo-political units smaller than a community (such as a school) have limitations for evaluat-ing effects on incidence or prevalence due to substantial in-migration and out-migration and the stability of estimates. Units larger than communities make experimental evaluations of interventions difficult, especially if one is attempting to employ randomized controlled trials.

A Goal for Community Practices Relevant to Childrearing

At the most general level, the goal of preventive practice in communities could be stated as ensuring that the largest possible proportion of young people arrive at adulthood with all of the skills and motivations they need to be healthy and succeed financially and socially. Thus, they would need to be able to maintain gainful employment, develop and maintain long-lasting friendships, and establish and maintain family relationships that are full of nurturance and relatively lacking in strife and abuse. And, they would not smoke cigarettes, drink in excess, fail to exercise, abuse illicit drugs, engage in sexual behavior that risks unwanted pregnancy or sexu-ally transmitted disease.

Fundamental Influences on Youth Development

In a sense, the nurturance of happy and successful children is not compli-
cated. One can describe the features of a nurturing environment in terms
of a small number of generic descriptors. Children and adolescents will engage in the behaviors that will further develop their skill and avoid risky or
unhealthy behavior if that behavior is richly reinforced and behavior that
puts them at risk for problems is made costly to them through the provision
of consistent, mild, negative consequences. In addition, they need frequent
and appropriate models of relevant skills and opportunities for reinforced
practice of those skills. Relevant skills include not only the obvious academic skills, but also skills for getting along with others. Opportunities to
engage in problematic or risky behavior need to be minimized.

The child or adolescent's biological capacity to engage in and be reinforced for appropriate behavior also must be considered. Numerous biological factors have been identified that make it more likely that a child
will be unable to engage in the behavior needed to succeed in his or her
current setting and will thereby be unable to develop the repertoire needed
to succeed later on (Fishbein, 2000).

Thus, the things that communities can do to ensure that the largest
possible proportion of children develop to their potential can be organized
into seven imperatives. These are:

(a) Prevent biological insult that puts children and adolescents at risk for the
    development of problems;
(b) Richly reinforce skilled social, cognitive, and physical behavior;
(c) Minimize opportunities to engage in problematic behavior;
(d) Consistently provide mild negative consequences for problematic behav-
    ior that does occur;
(e) Monitor young people's activities to ensure maximal opportunities for
    desirable behavior and minimal opportunities for problematic behavior
    and to enable effective consequences to be delivered;
(f) Provide numerous models in the media and real life of skilled behavior
    and effective instruction in needed social and cognitive or academic skills;
    and
(g) Ensure effective instructional practices are used to help young people
    maximize their academic and cognitive skills.

Biglan (1995) provides a detailed description of the evidence in support of the importance of these conditions.

Most of the empirically evaluated interventions to prevent youth problem behavior that are described in this book have their effect through one

or more of these mechanisms. Most of the interventions developed thus far have focused on affecting young people through their school or their family. However, there are other avenues to influence young people, including media, neighborhoods, and organizations relevant to young people.

The following sections describe how each of these influences on youth development might be optimized through programs and policies focused on families, schools, neighborhood and community organizations, and the media.

Preventing Biological Dysfunction

Fishbein (2000) has provided a useful summary of the ways in which children's development is affected by neurobiological conditions. Some of the factors are, of course, genetic. However, she points out that whether a particular genotype results in the development of problematic behavioral patterns depends, in part, on whether the environment has the other conditions described below. Moreover, there are numerous environmental events that compromise neurobiological functions.

Fetal development is harmed by inadequate nutrition, the use of drugs (especially tobacco, alcohol, and cocaine), and the mother's experience of stressful events. The consequences of such prenatal trauma include impaired cognitive function and patterns of irritability that put children at risk for the development of conduct disorders. Similarly, perinatal complications including prematurity and infectious disease put infants at risk for developing antisocial behavior (Piquero & Tibbetts, 1999). Therefore, it is not surprising that nurse visitation to poor, single teenage mothers has been shown to prevent the development of behavior problems and to improve cognitive development (Olds, 1997; Olds, Henderson et al., 1998; Olds, Pettitt et al., 1998). One of the most carefully evaluated programs involves the provision of nurse visitations to poor, single, teenage mothers (Olds, Henderson et al., 1998). The visits begin before the baby is born and continue for two years after birth. The nurses assist mothers to maintain good health practices during the prenatal period, including quitting smoking, eating well, and having prenatal medical care. Following birth, the nurses help mothers develop nurturing childcare. The program has been shown to reduce prenatal smoking, to delay the incidence of a second pregnancy, increase mothers' employment and earnings, and reduce child behavior problems among their children. Analysis of the savings that result from this program (compared with not having such a program) indicate that it can reduce government welfare costs by $24,694, increase mother's income by $1,010, and reduce public costs through crime prevention by

$5,062 per teenage mother. Programs of the sort described by Olds should be a fundamental component of every community's plan for preventing youth problems.

Postnatal development is also affected by the child's environment (Fishbein, 2000). Mother-child interactions affect neural development, which has implications for both children's cognitive capacity and their cooperative behavior. Both neglectful and abusive patterns of parental behavior can perturb the development of the cerebral cortex and affect key neurotransmitters including dopamine and serotonin. Abnormalities in these transmitter systems have been linked to an increased risk of both drug abuse and antisocial behavior (Fishbein, 1998). Harmful effects of trauma on neurobiology have also been shown for adolescents. They include disruptions in neurotransmitter activity and metabolism that have been associated with an increased likelihood of problems with alcohol and antisocial behavior.

Thus, it appears vital from a biological perspective that communities do what they can to ensure that families and other child-care providers minimize aversive or traumatic conditions that can permanently compromise children's biological capacity to develop successfully. Fortunately, there has been considerable research identifying family interventions and preschool programs that can minimize traumatic or stressful conditions while maximizing more positive ones described here (Biglan, 1995).

Reinforcement of Desirable Behavior

Perhaps the single most important principle developed by psychologists in the 20th century is that behavior is shaped and maintained by reinforcing consequences. The development of a child's skills and abilities results from reinforcing the consequences their fledgling behaviors achieve both from the inanimate environment and from parents, siblings, peers, teachers, and other adults.

Close inspection of most of the programs that have been developed to treat or prevent child and adolescent problems will show that one of their key components is an effort to increase positive reinforcement for desirable behavior. Perhaps the most extensively evaluated and empirically supported parenting interventions are the behavioral parenting skills programs (Taylor & Biglan, 1998; Wahler & Dumas, 1989). All versions of these programs, whether for children or adolescents, teach parents to use extrinsic reward to motivate behavior that the young person is having difficulty developing and to increase their rate of praise of desired behavior (e.g., Irvine, Biglan, Smolkowski, Metzler, & Ary, 1999; Webster-Stratton &

Herbert, 1994). In classrooms in which teachers praise, reward, and attend to children when they are on-task, cooperative, or well behaved, these behaviors occur more frequently. Indeed, problem behavior in middle school can be prevented by high levels of reinforcement for appropriate behavior in first grade (Kellam & Anthony, 1998; Kellam, Ling, Merisca, Brown, & Ialongo, 1998). In short, it is in the interest of families, schools, and communities to richly reinforce children's desirable behavior.

The widespread use of reinforcement has been impeded by common erroneous assertions that rewarding children's behavior would undermine their intrinsic motivation to do things (Cameron & Pierce, 1994). Our communities could do far more to become places in which children's desirable behavior, as well as good parenting and teaching practices, receive more recognition, praise, and reward than they do now. Examples of such efforts are available. In the Community Builders program, a community-wide intervention that helped to reduce middle school problem behavior (Metzler, Biglan, Rusby, & Sprague, 2001), community businesses donated numerous prizes to be used to reward appropriate social behavior and the radio and newspaper provided frequent recognition of young people's successes.

We are not suggesting simply that the community start a system of annual or monthly recognition of outstanding students. Such reinforcement would be too infrequent to make much difference and it would probably involve providing added recognition to young people who were already successful and getting a good deal of reinforcement. Rather, communities need to find innovative ways to praise and recognize prosocial behavior of every child on a daily basis. That might seem unrealistic, but in Dennis Embry's innovative Peacebuilders program that inspired our Community Builders intervention, it has been done (Embry, Flannery, Vazsonyi, Powell, & Atha, 1996). He organized several communities to provide daily recognition of one child from each elementary school in the city on the evening television news.

Another empirically evaluated example of a way that community organizations can provide incentives to young people is the Quantum Opportunity Program. It involves offering monetary incentives as well as learning opportunities to at-risk young people. The program has been shown to increase high school completion and college enrollment and substantially decrease arrest rate among participants (Taggart, 1995).

Thus, communities should be encouraged and assisted in substantially increasing the reinforcement that parents, teachers, police, child-care workers, and other young people provide for the behavior of every child or adolescent in the community. Doing so will prevent problems while contributing to positive youth development.

Minimizing Opportunities for Problem Behavior

Although it might seem that young people cannot engage in problem behaviors unless they have opportunities to do so, there has been little systematic development of approaches to reducing opportunities for problem behavior. Richardson (1981) has shown that young adolescents are significantly more likely to experiment with alcohol, tobacco, and other drugs if they are at home or at a friend's house when there are no adults around. Similarly, it is clear that easy access to substances is associated with greater use (Forster, Wolfson, Murray, Wagenaar, & Claxton, 1997; Holder, 1998). In schools, aggressive social behavior is more likely where adult supervision is minimal, such as on the playground and in the hallways (Walker, Colvin, & Ramsey, 1995). Communities would benefit from pinpointing the settings that provide opportunities for problem behavior so that they can alter them.

Researchers on alcohol and its attendant problems have done the most promising work in this area. There are now numerous studies showing that alcohol-related car crashes among young people can be significantly reduced through laws and regulations that make alcohol less accessible (Holder, 1994). The laws include increases in the legal drinking age and efforts to increase enforcement of restrictions on underage sales.

Similar research on reducing access to tobacco indicates that communities that adopt and enforce ordinances that restrict illegal sales of tobacco to young people can bring about a significant reduction in the prevalence of adolescent tobacco use (Forster et al., 1998; Jason, Berk, Schnopp-Wyatt, & Talbot, 1999). Recently, suggestive evidence is accumulating about the benefit of provisional driver's licenses for teenagers (Leaf & Preusser, 2000). Such licenses restrict the times at which 16-year-olds can drive and prohibit them from driving with other teenagers (Beck, 2000). The approach is based on clear evidence that youth are more likely to be in car crashes when there are other teens in the car or when they are driving late at night.

Presumably there are other things that communities can do to reduce the opportunities for young people to engage in problem behavior. Given the evidence that early adolescent experimentation with drugs and risky sexual behavior is most likely to occur in the afternoon at homes where young people meet without adult supervision, communities could increase the availability of supervised recreation activities after school for children and adolescents. To date we are unaware of any experimental evaluations of the effects of communities providing afterschool activities on the rates of problem behaviors.

Communities could reduce opportunities for problem behavior in many other ways. They could routinely identify public places were young people congregate and make sure that there is a sufficient adult presence to discourage problem behavior.

There is recent evidence that crime can be prevented through redesign of environments or "target hardening." A review of 16 studies by Casteel and Peek (2000) concluded that multicomponent programs of environmental redesign reduced robbery rates from 30 to 84%.

Providing Consistent Mild Negative Consequences for Unwanted Behavior

Numerous experimental and correlational studies in economics and psychology show that when one increases the cost of a behavior, the behavior becomes less likely (Biglan, 1995). The judicious use of consistent mild negative consequences can do much to ensure successful development. Unfortunately, in all venues involving young people, our society makes the same two mistakes: we fail to consistently provide small, effective consequences for minor inappropriate behaviors that lead to more serious problems, but we provide harsh consequences once problematic behavior occurs.

Programs for parents of children or adolescents with behavior problems assist parents in consistently providing mild negative consequences for a small number of behaviors that the parents consider inappropriate. Typical consequences are time out, loss of privileges, and small work chores. At the same time, the programs help parents decrease criticism and displays of anger and give up the use of very harsh penalties such as grounding for a month. Such harsh and inconsistent discipline actually contributes to aggressive and antisocial behavior (Patterson, Reid, & Dishion, 1992).

Similarly, effective behavior management systems in schools employ a small number of clear rules, provide mild consequences for rule violation (for example, an hour of community service for getting into a fight), but place their greatest emphasis on increasing opportunities and reinforcement for prosocial behavior (Horner & Day, 1991; Mayer, 1998; Metzler, Biglan, Rusby, & Sprague, 2001; Walker et al., 1995). Implementation of these systems typically *reduce* the amount of negative consequences delivered to young people because schools that have many rules and make great use of punishment actually have higher levels of vandalism and behavior problems (Mayer, 1998).

Our juvenile justice system provides the most egregious example of the excessive use of punishment. Typically, there are no consequences for minor juvenile offenses, such as possession of tobacco or alcohol. It is said that the system does not have the wherewithal to handle the high volume of these offenses. So, they tend to be overlooked. Once a young person begins to exhibit more serious criminal behavior, however, severe punishment is liberally applied. Increasingly, juvenile offenders are being remanded to adult courts and are receiving hard jail time. The juvenile justice system might deter more crime if it set up a system to ensure that young people reliably receive mild negative consequence for specific problem behaviors that, if not curtailed, are likely to lead to more serious offenses. Peer courts have been established in some places in order to provide such consequences for minor criminal offenses that are too costly to remand to juvenile courts. However, their efficacy appears not to have been tested in experimental studies.

Three things should be stressed about any effort to increase negative consequences for problem behavior, however. First, there is currently no experimental evidence on the merit of this approach. Implementation of these approaches should only be done if they can be experimentally evaluated. Second, care must be taken to prevent escalation of punishment for offenses. Harsh punishment may do more harm than good. For example, simply requiring restitution for an act of vandalism may be all that is necessary to deter further acts. Third, many efforts to deal with minor delinquency have backfired because they "widened the net" and brought young people into the criminal justice system who would not otherwise have been contacted by the system. Interventions that put these young people in further contact with other offenders have been shown to increase subsequent offending (Dishion, McCord, & Poulin, 1999).

In general, it seems better for those concerned with preventing youth problem behaviors to try to shift the emphasis from punishing serious offenses to providing many opportunities and reinforcement for appropriate behavior and consistent mild consequences for a small number of misbehaviors that are predictive of later more serious crime. As a matter of both humane treatment and effective childrearing, we should aim to ensure that the every child receives a far greater number of positive consequences for desirable behavior than negative consequences for undesired behavior.

Another type of mild negative consequence is the financial cost of a behavior. Increases in the cost of alcohol, through increased taxation, have been shown to decrease the use of these substances (Holder & Blose, 1987). In the case of tobacco, increased tobacco taxes have been shown to lower the prevalence of adolescent smoking (U.S. Department of Health and Human Services, 1994). Increased taxation may be the simplest and most cost-effective step that can be taken to deter the use of these substances, since it does not cost money. Indeed, some of the tax proceeds can be earmarked for other preventive efforts. The trick is to generate public support for such measures in the face of the opposition that will come from tobacco and alcohol interests. Strategies for overcoming such obstacles are available (e.g., Biglan, 1995).

Monitoring Young People's Activities

Most of what we know about the value of monitoring young people's activities comes from studies of parental monitoring. Parents who know what their child or adolescent is doing each day are less likely to have children who are associating with deviant peers and engaging in diverse problem behaviors (Biglan & Smolkowski, 2002; Dishion & McMahon, 1998). Presumably, parents who know what their children are doing are able to detect when the child is drifting into activities that might pose a risk. They are able to reduce opportunities for problems by steering their children away from risky situations; at the same time they are able to provide positive reinforcement for desired behavior and effective negative consequences when violations of parental rules or expectations occur.

In schools, the ongoing monitoring of children's academic progress is an essential feature of effective instruction (Becker, 1986). That is, teachers should be assessing at least weekly whether students are gaining the targeted skills so that they can adjust their teaching strategies to ensure academic progress. Students' social progress is generally not monitored unless the child is engaging in high levels of aggressive or disruptive behavior. Increased monitoring of social interactions in playground settings could help to prevent the development of some aggressive behavior among elementary school students if it prompted teachers and other school personnel to promote prosocial behavior and reduce aggressive behavior. It would seem that communities could increase the monitoring of young people that occurs in public settings through community policing and the provision of supervised recreation, which facilitates monitoring. However, the latter type of monitoring would need to be done to pinpoint settings that have high potential for problem behavior, so that those settings could be changed. It should not be done simply to increase surveillance of young people and opportunities for punishing them.

Modeling and Media

From infancy, children are enormously skilled in learning by observing models (Bandura, 1962). Children's verbal development hinges on their being exposed to thousands of instances of other's verbal behavior. Large differences in the number of modeled verbal behaviors have been observed in comparisons of middle class and working class families and it has been suggested that this may help to account for the greater verbal facility of middle class children (Risley & Hart, 1968). It has also been demonstrated in numerous experimental studies that children can imitate complex behavior of others and they are especially likely to do so, if they observe that the modeled behavior is reinforced (Bandura, 1962; Biglan, 1995).

Thus, communities should be concerned to ensure that children and adolescents are exposed to numerous reinforced models of skilled behavior, including academic activities, cooperation, supportive behavior, and so on. They should be similarly concerned that models of aggressive or otherwise antisocial behavior be kept to a minimum.

Unfortunately, most communities in the United States are failing to prevent models of antisocial behavior from flooding the lives of their children and adolescents. Despite the fact that it is well established that exposure to models of aggressive behavior increases child and adolescent aggressive behavior (Jason & Hanaway, 1997), many young people are exposed to a daily diet of models of aggression on television and in video games. Although clearly not every child becomes more aggressive as a result of viewing such models, a subset of children is affected. Moreover, regular exposure to such models inures young people to violence in ways that may make it harder for our society to become mobilized to create the conditions for a more peaceful civic life (Jason & Hanaway, 1997).

Finding ways to reduce children's exposure to media violence or the effects of viewing it should be a high priority for researchers and policymakers. Parents are the main barriers to young people's exposure to such models. Movie theaters and video rental stores might be influenced to do a better job of preventing young people access to the most egregious examples of violence. However, even PG rated movies can contain much violence and most everything is available on cable stations. There has been little research showing that parents can successfully prevent their children from being exposed to problematic models of aggressive behavior (Jason & Hanaway, 1997).

It also may be possible to inoculate children to the effects of viewing violence by teaching them to distinguish between media depictions and real life (Huesmann, Eron, Klein, Brice, & Fischer, 1983). However, we are a long way from implementing such teaching on a broad scale.

Then there is the influence of media in marketing products that harm young people. There is now substantial evidence that tobacco-marketing practices influence vulnerable adolescents to take up smoking (Pierce, Choi, Gilpin, Farkas, & Merritt, 1996; Pierce & Gilpin, 1995; Pucci & Siegel, 1999a, 1999b; Saffer & Chaloupka, 2000; Unger, Johnson, & Rohrbach, 1995; While, Kelly, Huang, & Charlton, 1996). The appealing images of smokers that are presented in advertising and promotional activities influence many young people to think that they can have desired qualities such as maturity, popularity, fun, and toughness through smoking. Similar processes occur for alcohol use (Holder, 1994).

Recently, Saffer & Chaloupka (2000) showed that a complete ban on advertising of cigarettes could significantly reduce adolescent onset of smoking. We may be far from the enactment of such a policy, but its value should be the subject of increased public discussion.

Effective Instruction

For more than 20 years, the key features of effective instructional practices have been understood. Becker (1986) provided a useful summary of them:

1. Objectives are specified.
2. Preskills are tested to ensure appropriate placement.
3. Procedures are developed to motivate and engage the student in active learning.
4. [Instruction is designed] that teaches the targeted objectives effectively and efficiently.
5. Differential time is allowed for different students to reach mastery.
6. Ungraded, frequent testing is provided to monitor progress.
7. Corrective-remedial procedures are provided if an approach fails.
8. Adequate practice is provided to master sub-skills.
9. There is testing for longer-term mastery of objectives.

Sadly, the educational establishment in most states and communities has failed to adopt the most effective practices (e.g., Hirsch, 1996). This appears to be changing. For example, effective approaches to reading instruction—perhaps the most critical skill for academic success—were recently summarized by a blue ribbon federal panel (National Reading Panel, 2000). Their recommendations guided federal legislation that is designed to promote more effective reading instruction throughout the nation.

Efforts to inform the business community about empirically supported teaching practices have encouraged the adoption of such practices (Biglan, Mrazek, Carnine, & Flay, in press). Given the long history of fads and unevaluated teaching practices in schools, community leaders who are concerned about the successful development of the children in their community should not leave it to educators to decide on educational practice until they are satisfied that research-based instructional practices are being employed and students' progress is being carefully monitored.

The Need for a System for Monitoring Child and Adolescent Well-Being

Thus far, I have described practices that would ensure the successful development of most children and adolescents. However, there is another practice that communities should adopt if they want to ensure the success of their children. It is the careful monitoring of child and adolescent well-being. Consider that the management of other aspects of our society such as our economy and our health are guided by detailed and ongoing measurement of key indicators. Why should we not demand the same care in ensuring that our children are developing successfully?

Systems for monitoring child and adolescent well-being are becoming more common. For example, Pollard, Hawkins, and Arthur (1999) have developed a set of measures that they are using to help communities in at least six states assess adolescent problem behavior and the level of risk and protective factors that have been shown to influence development. Profiles of communities' strengths and weaknesses are available to guide what the communities do to improve outcomes for their young people.

The further development and dissemination of such systems should bring us to the point where gradual improvements in child and adolescent development occur as communities retain practices that the data suggest are working and drop or modify those that do not seem to be of value.

Toward More Effective Communities

This book has delineated a wealth of opportunities for communities to improve outcomes for children and adolescents. Preceding chapters summarize programs and policies that have been shown to affect one or more of the most common and costly problems of young people. The present chapter has described the key components of those programs in a way that could facilitate more extensive use of these practices in efforts to support successful youth development.

Therein lie the ingredients for more effective childrearing in communities. What will be needed to translate this knowledge into more successful communities? One thing is the widespread communication of this knowledge to all of the policymakers and program directors at the federal, state, and local levels able to affect practices in communities. Another is the increased coordination among these actors. Most of the problems of childhood and adolescence are interrelated and arise from the same set of biological and environmental influences. The organizations that have responsibility for one or more aspects of youth development are not yet organized in light of these facts. It is imperative that they develop additional coordinated and comprehensive approaches to youth development to reflect these facts.

Research in the last forty years has brought us to the point where communities can be far more successful than they currently are in assuring that every child becomes a healthy, happy, and productive adult. It is time now for us to evolve the childrearing practices of every community so that the potential of this knowledge becomes a reality.

References

Bandura, A. (1962). Social learning through imitation. *Proceedings of the Nebraska Symposium on Motivation*, 211–269.

Beck, K.H. (2000, June). *Parental influence on adolescent driving risk.* Paper presented at the annual meeting of the Society for Prevention Research, Montreal, Quebec, Canada.

Becker, W.C. (1986). *Applied psychology for teachers.* Chicago: Science Research Associates.

Biglan, A. (1995). *Changing cultural practices: A contextualist framework for intervention research.* Reno, NV: Context Press.

Biglan, A., Mrazek, P., Carnine, D.W., & Flay, B.R. (in press). The integration of research and practice in the prevention of youth problem behaviors. *American Psychologist.*

Biglan, A., & Smolkowski, K. (2002). Intervention effects on adolescent drug use and critical influences on the development of problem behavior. In D.B. Kandel (Ed.), *Stages and pathways of drug involvement: Examining the Gateway Hypothesis.* New York: Cambridge University Press.

Cameron, J., & Pierce, W.D. (1994). Reinforcement, reward, and intrinsic motivation: A meta-analysis. *Review of Educational Research, 64,* 363–423.

Casteel C., & Peek, A.C. (2000). Effectiveness of crime prevention through environmental design (CPTED) in reducing robberies. *American Journal of Preventive Medicine, 18,* 99–115

Dishion, T.J., McCord, J., & Poulin, F. (1999). When interventions harm: Peer groups and problem behavior. *American Psychologist, 54,* 755–764.

Dishion, T.J. & McMahon, R.J. (1998). Parental monitoring and the prevention of problem behavior: A conceptual and empirical reformulation. In R.S. Ashery, E.B. Robertson &

K.L. Kumpfer (Eds.), *Drug abuse prevention through family interventions. NIDA Monograph 177* (pp. 229–59). Rockville, MD: U.S. Dept. of Health & Human Services, NIH.

Embry, D.E., Flannery, D., Vazsonyi, A., Powell, K., & Atha, H. (1996). Peace-Builders: A theoretically driven, school-based model for early violence prevention. *American Journal of Preventive Medicine, 22*, 91–100.

Fishbein, D.H. (1998). Differential susceptibility to comorbid drug abuse and violence. *Journal of Drug Issues, 28*, 859–90.

Fishbein, D.H. (2000). *The science, treatment, and prevention of antisocial behaviors. Application to the criminal justice system.* Kingston, NJ: Civic Research Institute.

Forster, J.L., Murray, D.M., Wolfson, M., Blaine, T.M., Wagenaar, A.C., & Hennrikus, D.J. (1998). The effects of community policies to reduce youth access to tobacco. *American Journal of Public Health, 88*, 1193–98.

Forster, J.L., Wolfson, M., Murray, D.M., Wagenaar, A.C., & Claxton, A.J. (1997). Perceived and measured availability of tobacco to youth in fourteen Minnesota communities: The TPOP Study. *American Journal of Preventive Medicine, 13*, 167–74.

Hawkins, J.D., Catalano, R.F., & Miller, J.Y. (1992). Risk and protective factors for alcohol and other drug problems in adolescence and early adulthood: Implications for substance abuse prevention. *Psychological Bulletin, 112*, 64–105.

Hirsch, E.D.J. (1996). *The schools we need and why we don't have them.* New York: Doubleday.

Holder, H. (1994). Mass communication as an essential aspect of community prevention to reduce alcohol-involved traffic crashes. *Alcohol, Drugs, and Driving, 10*, 295–307.

Holder, H.D. (1998). *Alcohol and the community: A systems approach to prevention.* Cambridge: Cambridge University Press.

Holder, H.D., & Blose, J.O. (1987). Reduction of community alcohol problems: Computer simulation experiments in three countries. *Journal of Studies on Alcohol, 48*, 124–35.

Horner, R.H., & Day, H.M. (1991). The effects of response efficiency on functionally equivalent competing behaviors. *Journal of Applied Behavior Analysis, 24*, 719–32.

Huesmann, L.R., Eron, L.D., Klein, R., Brice, P., & Fischer, P. (1983). Mitigating the imitation of aggressive behaviors by changing children's attitudes about media violence. *Journal of Personality and Social Psychology, 44*, 899–910.

Irvine, A.B., Biglan, A., Smolkowski, K., Metzler, C.W., & Ary, D.V. (1999). The effectiveness of a parenting skills program for parents of middle school students in small communities. *Journal of Consulting and Clinical Psychology, 67*, 811–25.

Jason, L.A., Berk, M., Schnopp-Wyatt, D.L., & Talbot, B. (1999). Effects of enforcement of youth access laws on smoking prevalence. *American Journal of Community Psychology, 27*, 143–60.

Jason, L.A., & Hanaway, L.K. (1997). *Remote control. A sensible approach to kids, TV, and the new electronic media.* Sarasota, FL: Professional Resource Press.

Kellam, S.G., & Anthony, J.C. (1998). Targeting early antecedents to prevent tobacco smoking: Findings from an epidemiologically based randomized field trial. *American Journal of Public Health, 88*, 1490–95.

Kellam, S.G., Ling, X., Merisca, R., Brown, C.H., & Ialongo, N. (1998). The effect of the level of aggression in the first grade classroom on the course and malleability of aggressive behavior into middle school. *Development & Psychopathology, 10*, 165–85.

Leaf, W.A., & Preusser, D.F. (2000, June). *Effects of components of graduated licensing.* Paper presented at the annual meeting of the Society for Prevention, Montreal, Quebec, Canada.

Mayer, G.R. (1998) *Do educators contribute to student antisocial behavior?* Unpublished manuscript, California State University at Los Angeles.

Metzler, C.W., Biglan, A., Rusby, J.C, & Sprague, J. (2001). Evaluation of a comprehensive behavior management program to improve school-wide positive behavior support. *Education and Treatment of Children, 24*(4), 448–79.

National Reading Panel (2000, December 13). *National Reading Panel: Teaching children to read: An evidence-based assessment of the scientific research literature on reading and its implications for reading instruction.* Retrieved December 13, 2001, from *http://www.nichd.nih.gov/publications/nrp/smallbook.htm*

Olds, D. (1997). The prenatal early infancy project: Preventing child abuse and neglect in the context of promoting maternal and child health. In *Child abuse: New directions in prevention and treatment across the lifespan* (pp. 130–154). Thousand Oaks, CA: Sage.

Olds, D.L., Henderson, C.R., Jr., Kitzman, H.J., Eckenrode, J., Cole, R.E., & Tatelbaum, R. (1998). The promise of home visitation: Results of two randomized trials. *Journal of Community Psychology, 26,* 5–21.

Olds, D.L., Pettitt, L.M., Robinson, J., Henderson, C.R., Jr., Eckenrode, J., Kitzman, H., et al. (1998). Reducing risks for antisocial behavior with a program of prenatal and early childhood home visitation. *Journal of Community Psychology, 26,* 65–83.

Patterson, G.R., Reid, J.B., & Dishion, T.J. (1992). *Antisocial boys: A social interactional approach, Vol. 4.* Eugene, OR: Castalia.

Pierce, J.P., Choi, W.S., Gilpin, E.A., Farkas, A.J., & Merritt, R.K. (1996). Validation of susceptibility as a predictor of which adolescents take up smoking in the United States. *Health Psychology, 15,* 355–61.

Pierce, J.P., & Gilpin, E.A. (1995). A historical analysis of tobacco marketing and the uptake of smoking by youth in the United States: 1890–1977. *Health Psychology, 14,* 500–08.

Piquero, A., & Tibbetts, S. (1999). The impact of pre/perinatal disturbances and disadvantaged familial environment in predicting criminal offending. *Studies on Crime and Crime Prevention, 8(1),* 52–70

Pollard, J.A., Hawkins, J.D., & Arthur, M.W. (1999). Risk and protection: Are both necessary to understand diverse behavioral outcomes in adolescence? *Social Work Research, 23*(3), 145–58.

Pucci, L., & Siegel, M. (1999a). Exposure to brand-specific cigarette advertising in magazines and its impact on youth smoking. *Preventive Medicine, 29,* 313–20.

Pucci L.G,. & Siegel, M. (1999b). Features of sales promotion in cigarette magazine advertisements, 1980–1993: An analysis of youth exposure in the United States. *Tobacco Control, 8,* 29–36.

Richardson, G.E. (1981). Educational imagery: A missing link in decision-making. *Journal of School Health,* 560–64.

Risley, T.R., & Hart, B. (1968). Developing correspondence between the non-verbal and verbal behavior of preschool children. *Journal of Applied Behavior Analysis, 1,* 267–81.

Saffer, H., & Chaloupka, F. (2000). The effect of tobacco advertising bans on tobacco consumption. *Journal of Health Economics, 19,* 1117–37.

Taggart, R. (1995). *Quantum Opportunity Program.* Philadelphia: Opportunities Industrialization Centers of America.

Taylor, T.K., & Biglan, A. (1998). Behavioral family interventions: A review for clinicians and policymakers. *Clinical Child and Family Psychology Review, 1,* 41–60.

U. S. Department of Health and Human Services. (1994). *Preventing tobacco use among young people: A report of the Surgeon General.* Atlanta, Georgia: Author.

Unger, J.B., Johnson, C.A., & Rohrbach, L.A. (1995). Recognition and liking of tobacco and alcohol advertisements among adolescent. *Preventive Medicine, 24,* 461–66.

Wahler, R.G., & Dumas, J.E. (1989). Attentional problems in dysfunctional mother-child interactions: An interbehavioral model. *Psychological Bulletin, 105,* 116–30.

Walker, H.M., Colvin, G., & Ramsey, E. (1995). *Antisocial behavior in school: Strategies and best practices.* Pacific Grove, CA: Brooks/Cole.

Webster-Stratton, C., & Herbert, M. (1994). *Troubled families—problem children: Working with parents: A collaborative process.* Chichester, England: John Wiley & Sons.

While, D., Kelly, S., Huang, W., & Charlton, A. (1996). Cigarette advertising and onset of smoking in children: Questionnaire survey. *British Medical Journal, 313,* 398–99.

Chapter 7

Conclusions and Recommendations

Herbert J. Walberg and Anthony Biglan

The authors of the foregoing chapters gathered together with other scholars and practicing professionals in education, social work, criminal justice, government policy, and related fields. They participated in a two-day conference in Washington, DC that was designed to formulate recommendations. Informed by the chapters, other scholarship, and a wide variety of professional experiences, they worked in small groups to set forth recommendations to improve children and youths' conditions and services for the prevention of such problems as alcohol, tobacco and illicit drug use, violence, and sexually transmitted diseases. The conferees achieved a considerable degree of consensus, but, of course, not every conferee would agree with all detailed points offered either by the groups or by our synthesis here. Still, the ideas expressed should offer constructive starting points for thinking about how conditions, policies, and practices for children and youth might best be improved at the local, state, and national levels.

Key Conclusions

The recommendations derive from three conclusions suggested in the foregoing chapters.

1. The first conclusion concerns the relationships among youth problem behavior and their causes. As each of the chapters noted, young people who have one of the problems under discussion are likely to have others. Moreover, it is striking how many of the risk factors for any one of the problems

163

are also risk factors for other problems. For example, early aggressive behavior, associations with deviant peers, and parent-child conflict make each of the other youth problems more likely. The development of more effective childrearing practices will need to be guided by these facts.

2. A second conclusion is that problematic and successful development depends on school, family, peer, and community factors. Preventing the problems addressed in this book and ensuring successful development requires that we address all of these factors.

3. Third, there is a substantial gap between science and practice. Although numerous scientifically validated programs and policies have been identified, they are not in widespread use, and it is still unclear how we can foster their widespread and effective implementation. With these considerations in mind, the group developed recommendations for what people in schools, communities, and state and national organizations can do to help prevent youth problems.

Schools

Schools should prepare children both academically and socially. Given that youth problem behaviors are very costly to society, contribute to academic failure, and generally stem from the same set of factors, schools should establish practices that ameliorate diverse youth problems by targeting the factors that lead to them. Comprehensive strategies are needed that identify and prevent early behavior problems, including aggressive social behavior, through effective behavior management and social skills training, as well as through programs that assist parents in supporting children's appropriate social behavior.

Also, school staff need to develop consistent ways of monitoring the social and behavioral development of their students. Annual assessments of problem behaviors are increasingly available. We should aim to enable all schools to conduct these assessments so that the school and community know the level of each problem behavior in the community and whether their efforts to prevent problems are effective.

If schools are to establish these practices, they will need clear summaries of the most effective practices. Decision makers at the state and local level should be informed about empirically supported practices for preventing problem behavior. Training is needed to provide teachers with the skills for effective behavior management and for identifying and intervening with aggressive children. Efforts will be needed to increase the pool of such skilled teachers both through increased training and through better retention of skilled people.

Communities

Effective childrearing is likely to flourish in communities that develop a clear and widely shared vision of the outcomes they want for their children and the practices that are likely to achieve those outcomes. Creating such a vision will foster collaborative relationships among teachers, parents, policymakers, and scientists and will inspire concerted effort to turn that vision into a reality.

Because diverse problems are interrelated and result from the same influences, community organizations should develop greater coordination so that funding supports the practices that are most likely to affect multiple problems. Effective childrearing will also be facilitated by systems for monitoring the well-being of children and adolescents and the status of risk and protective factors that affect youth development. Such monitoring can be built into the decision-making process of the community so that it guides attention to effective childrearing practices.

Children and youth programs are likely to be more effective if parents are involved in their planning and operation. Special help, however, is required for high-risk parents who may lack the skills to nurture their children's successful development.

Efforts to assist communities should not be top down. Although scientists and policymakers at the state and national level can provide critical information about childrearing, the best decisions about program planning and implementation are likely to be made at the community level and by parents. Community decision-making should engage the full range of professions serving children and youth. Requests for proposals and funding that require such an integrated approach may be the best way to promote integrated service delivery.

The practices that evolve for effective childrearing in communities will need to be predicated on an understanding that change in outcomes may take time. From the outset, there should be appropriate expectations regarding how much time may be needed for this change.

States and National Systems

A better system for articulating and disseminating information about effective practices is needed. Decision makers and the general public need to be educated about the programs and policies that have been shown to benefit youth. The diverse organizations that have been identifying "best practices" need to come together around a set of standards for which practices are ready for dissemination.

National-level organizations such as the National Institutes of Health, the Centers for Disease Control and Prevention, the Department of Justice, and the Department of Education need to develop integrated approaches to funding both programs and research. Comprehensive and coordinated strategies for preventing diverse youth problems are needed at the community level. Such strategies can help avoid duplication of effort and a failure to concentrate resources on the key influences that are common to diverse but related problems.

Research

The next generation of research should test comprehensive approaches to preventing diverse youth problems that target family, school, peer, neighborhood, and community influences on adolescent development. Research is needed on the effectiveness of programs and policies that have been shown to be of value in well-controlled studies, but have not necessarily been evaluated in the "real world" conditions of schools and communities. Research is also needed to evaluate strategies for effectively disseminating research-based programs, policies, and techniques. We still know little about how to help schools and communities make effective use of what has been developed by researchers. Both effectiveness and dissemination research will require a greater level of cooperation between researchers and practitioners. It would be beneficial to create a national network of researchers and school systems that implement and experimentally evaluate empirically supported practices. A national network might best evaluate practices devised in diverse schools and communities. In any case, partnerships among researchers and practitioners might clearly benefit them both as well as the youth they ultimately serve.

About the Editors

Anthony Biglan, Ph.D., is a Senior Scientist at Oregon Research Institute in Eugene, Oregon. He does research on the prevention of child and adolescent problem behavior and the childrearing practices that affect child and adolescent development. He is the author of the 1995 book, *Changing Cultural Practices: A Contextualist Framework for Intervention Research*, published by Context Press. Current work focuses on contextual analyses of childrearing practices in communities.

Dr. Biglan served on the Epidemiology & Prevention Review Committee for the National Institute on Drug Abuse (NIDA) and on Review Committees for the National Institutes of Health (NIH). He is on the editorial boards of four national journals and consults with the Office of National Drug Control Policy. He is a board member of the Society of Prevention Research and co-chairs its Prevention Science Advocacy Committee.

Herbert J. Walberg, Ph.D., is University Scholar and Emeritus Professor of Education and Psychology at the University of Illinois at Chicago and Distinguished Visiting Fellow at Stanford University (1999–2004). Dr. Walberg has served on numerous boards-as well as national and international advisory committees. He has also written and edited more than 55 books and written about 350 articles on topics such as educational effectiveness and exceptional human accomplishments. Among his latest books are the *International Encyclopedia of Educational Evaluation* and *Psychology and Educational Practice*. He is also a fellow of five academic societies including the American Association for the Advancement of Science, the International Academy of Education, and the American Psychological Society.

About the Authors

Henry D. Anaya, Ph.D., is a Health Research Scientist affiliated with the United States Veteran's Administration Health Services Research and Development (HSR&D) Center for Excellence in Los Angeles. Previously, Dr. Anaya served with the UCLA/Neuropsychiatric Institute Center for Community Health as Associate Director of the UCLA Center for HIV Identification, Prevention, and Treatment Services (CHIPTS). Dr. Anaya's areas of concentration are race and ethnic relations, social stratification and health disparities, HIV/AIDS research, community-based health interventions, and health and educational policy evaluation. In addition to this chapter, he is author of a theoretical paper on the permeability of racial and ethnic boundary formation, and is currently completing a manuscript examining childhood sexual abuse among youth living with HIV. His current research examines quality of care interventions among HIV-positive veterans within the Veteran's Administration healthcare system—the largest provider of health care for HIV-positive individuals in the United States. He has previously served as an evaluation consultant to local and federal governments, and continues to consult on both regional and national evaluation projects, the most current of which examines disparities in health care among Native Americans. Dr. Anaya received his Ph.D. in sociology from Stanford University in 1999.

Susan M. Cantwell, J.D., is Director of Publications for the Center for Community Health in the Neuropsychiatric Institute, University of California, Los Angeles. She earned a Bachelor of Arts degree in government and psychology from the University of Notre Dame and a Juris Doctorate degree, with an emphasis on criminal law in child and family protection, from California Western School of Law. As a certified graduate of an interdisciplinary program on child abuse and neglect in law school, Dr. Cantwell authored two manuscripts that focus on the ramifications of the justice system on children. She is involved in all levels of manuscript preparation and submission for the Center, as well as the management, coordination, and preparation of presentation materials. Dr. Cantwell is interested in HIV and mental health policy research, especially in the field of implications for children and families. In addition, she is interested in exploring and developing strategies that will bring interventions to scale.

Philip A. Fisher, Ph.D., is a Research Scientist at the Oregon Social Learning Center (OSLC) in Eugene, Oregon. He is particularly interested in prevention of antisocial behaviors in the early years of life. Dr. Fisher is a Principal Investigator on the *Early Intervention Foster Care Project* (EIFC), a five-year randomized trial funded by the National Institute on Mental Health (NIMH) to test the effectiveness of a preventive intervention for maltreated preschool-aged foster children. The intervention incorporates many of the elements of OSLC's Treatment Foster Care program for adolescents, and adds additional components such as a focus on developmental delays and a home visitation model of service delivery that are designed to meet the needs of children in this age group. The research being conducted on the EIFC project examines how the intervention impacts multiple domains, including behavior, emotions, and neurobiology. Related to this project, Dr. Fisher is a co-investigator of an NIMH-funded network grant examining the effects of early experiences on glucocorticoid activity in the brain. Dr. Fisher is also involved in family-based prevention activities in American Indian communities. He is Principal Investigator of the *Indian Family Wellness* (IFW) project, a five-year study funded by the National Institute on Drug Abuse (NIDA) that involves collaboration with a tribal Head Start program. The IFW project is based on a tribal participatory research model. A major emphasis of IFW is the transfer of prevention research technology into the community, thereby allowing the tribe to set its own research agenda. Dr. Fisher also serves on a number of national advisory groups, including a NIDA workgroup of Native American researchers and scholars and a National Institutes of Health (NIH) study section that evaluates proposals for community-based interventions.

Brian Flay, Ph.D., is Distinguished Professor (Community Health Sciences in Public Health, as well as Psychology) at University of Illinois at Chicago. From 1987 to 1997, he was founding director of the Prevention Research Center. Dr. Flay has extensive experience with school-based research in the fields of smoking/drugs, AIDS, and violence prevention. He has held many PI positions on various drug and smoking prevention organizations. Dr. Flay is currently working with two NIDA-funded intervention projects.

The ABAN AYA Youth Project focuses on the prevention of high-risk behaviors such as drug use, unsafe sex, and violence in inner city African-
American schools and communities. The Positive Action Efficacy Study is a
randomized trial of the Positive Action program, a comprehensive K–6 program designed to improve student behavior and academic achievement.
Dr. Flay has served as a consultant for The Centers for Disease Control and
the Congressional Office of Technology Assessment, among many others,
and was a member of the National Research Panel on Evaluation of AIDS
Prevention Interventions (1999–2000). Dr. Flay is a Fellow of the Society of
Behavioral Medicine, the Society for Community Research and Action, and
the American Academy of Health Behavior. He has received national recognition for his research.

Sharon L. Foster, Ph.D., is a Professor in the Clinical Psychology doctoral
program at the California School of Professional Psychology at Alliant
International University in San Diego. Her many articles and book chapters address children's peer relations, parent-adolescent conflict, aggression in girls, and research methodology. She is coauthor of *Negotiating
Parent-Adolescent Conflict* (Guilford Press, 1989), which describes the development and evaluation of a treatment program for reducing acrimonious
parent-adolescent conflict. From 1996–2000, Dr. Foster edited the Clinical
Assessment Series for the Association for Advancement of Behavior
Therapy. She has been a member of editorial boards for some of the most
prestigious journals in her field, and has twice served as an Associate
Editor for rigorous methodologically oriented journals (*Behavioral Assessment, Journal of Consulting and Clinical Psychology*). Dr. Foster is currently
involved in projects related to the development, prevention, and treatment
of serious adolescent behavior problems, and to understanding the development of psychopathology—particularly aggression—in girls.

Mary Jane Rotheram-Borus, Ph.D., is a Professor of Psychiatry and
Director of the Center for HIV Identification, Prevention, and Treatment
Services and the Center for Community Health in the Neuropsychiatric
Institute, University of California, Los Angeles. Dr. Rotheram-Borus received her Ph.D. in Clinical Psychology from the University of Southern
California. Her research interests include HIV/AIDS prevention with adolescents, suicide among adolescents, homeless youths, assessment and
modification of children's social skills, ethnic identity, group processes,
and cross-ethnic interactions. Dr. Rotheram-Borus has received grants
from NIMH to study HIV prevention with adolescents and persons with
sexually transmitted diseases; to study interventions for children whose

parents have AIDS and for HIV-seropositive adolescents; and to examine national patterns of use, costs, outcomes, and need for children's and adolescents' mental health service programs.

Herbert H. Severson, Ph.D., is a Senior Scientist at Oregon Research Institute. Since 1978, he has been an investigator of NIH grants focused on development and evaluation of tobacco prevention and cessation. He has recently focused his research on evaluating smokeless tobacco (ST) cessation programs and school and community prevention programs that focus on improving parenting skills. He has conducted early studies on tobacco prevention and cessation.

Dr. Severson is an author of the 1986, 1994, and 2000 Surgeon General Reports and a 1994 report by the Institute of Medicine, *Growing Up Tobacco Free: Preventing Nicotine Addiction in Children and Youths*. In addition to over 100 articles in professional journals, he authored five books and over 20 video programs on tobacco use prevention. Dr. Severson has recently developed interactive CD-ROM cessation programs for adult smokeless tobacco users (*Chewer's Choice 2000*) and adolescents (*X-Chew Challenge 2000*), as well as a training program for oral health professionals (*Helping Your Patients Quit Tobacco 2001*).

Most recently, he has been funded to develop an Internet-delivered interactive program for smokeless tobacco cessation (ChewFree.com) and a parenting program to parents of Head Start children who are exhibiting high-risk behaviors (Parent Net). Dr. Severson is also working with the Department of Defense on a program for smokeless tobacco cessation using proactive phone counseling.

Robert A. Zucker, Ph.D., is a Professor of Psychology in the Departments of Psychiatry and Psychology at the University of Michigan, Ann Arbor. He also serves as Director of the University of Michigan Addiction Research Center (UMARC), Director of the Division of Substance Abuse in the Department of Psychiatry, and is Faculty Associate at the Institute for Social Research (Research Center for Group Dynamics). Dr. Zucker formerly served as President of the Division on Addictions of the American Psychological Association, one of the review editors for *Alcoholism: Clinical and Experimental Research*, as well as a consulting editor to four other scientific journals in the areas of substance abuse and developmental psychopathology. He serves as a member of the National Institute on Alcohol Abuse and Alcoholism (NIAAA) Advisory Council Subcomittee on College Drinking, and is a contributing author to the most recent NIAAA *Tenth Special Report to the U.S. Congress on Alcohol and Health*. The focus of Dr. Zucker's career research has been the lifespan etiology of substance abuse, with a special interest in the development and clinical course of alcoholism. For the past 18 years, Dr. Zucker has been the director of the Michigan-Michigan State University Longitudinal Study, and he directs UMARC's postdoctoral research training programs. He has authored over 180 publications and has edited nine books. Dr. Zucker is a diplomat of the American Board of Professional Psychology (ABPP) in clinical psychology.

Issues in Children's and Families' Lives

Series Editors:
Thomas P. Gullotta, *Child and Family Agency of Southeastern Connecticut, New London Connecticut;* **Herbert J. Walberg**, *University of Illinois at Chicago, Chicago Illinois;* **Roger P. Weisberg**, *University of Illinois at Chicago, Chicago, Illinois*

Series Mission

Using the collective resources of the Child and Family Agency of Southeastern Connecticut, one of the nation's leading family service agencies, and the University of Illinois at Chicago, one of the nation's outstanding universities, this series focuses attention on the pressing social and emotional problems facing young people and their families today.

Two publishing efforts are to be found within these volumes:

The first effort from the University of Illinois at Chicago Series on Children and Youth draws upon the multiple academic disciplines and the full range of human service professions to inform and stimulate policymakers and professionals that serve youth. The contributors use basic and applied research to uncover "the truth" and "the good" from such academic disciplines as psychology and sociology as well as such professions as education, medicine, nursing, and social work.

The second effort belongs to the Child and Family Hartman Scholars program. More than a decade in existence, this chosen group of scholars, practitioners, and advocates is formed yearly around a critical study area. This honored learning group analyzes, integrates, and critiques the clinical and research literature as it relates to the chosen theme and issues a volume that focuses on enhancing the physical, social, and emotional health of children and their families in relationship to that issue.

University Advisory Committee for
The University of Illinois at Chicago Series on
Children and Youth

177

National Advisory Committee for
The University of Illinois at Chicago Series on
Children and Youth

EDMUND W. GORDON
Professor Emeritus
Department of Psychology
Yale University
New Haven, CT

THOMAS P. GULLOTTA
Chief Executive Officer
Child and Family Agency of
    Southeastern Connecticut
New London, CT

ROBERT J. HAGGERTY
Professor of Pediatrics
School of Medicine and
    Dentistry
University of Rochester
Rochester, NY

IRVING HARRIS
Chairman of The Harris
    Foundation
Chicago, IL

ANNE C. PETERSEN
Senior Vice President for
    Programs
W. K. Kellogg Foundation
Battle Creek, MI

RUBY N. TAKANISHI
President
Foundation for Child Development
New York, NY

WILLIAM J. WILSON
Malcolm Wiener Professor of Social
    Policy
Malcolm Wiener Center for Social
    Policy
John F. Kennedy School of
    Government
Harvard University
Cambridge, MA

EDWARD ZIGLER
Sterling Professor of Psychology,
    Yale University;
Director,
Bush Center for Social Policy and
    Child Development
Yale University
New Haven, CT

179

Index

Postnatal development, 150
Pregnancies, teenage, 2, 116–117
Prenatal intervention, 13
 home visit intervention, 12, 18
Preschool-aged children
 antisocial behavior, interventions, 12–14
Problem behavior, childrearing and: see
  also Antisocial behavior
 consistent mild negative consequences
  for, 153–155
 minimizing opportunities for behavior,
  152–153
Problem Behavior Therapy, 38
Programs to Advance Teen Health: see
  Project PATH
Project Northland, 40, 100
Project PATH, 75, 101–102
Project Sixteen, 77, 101–102
Psychiatrically disturbed youth, sexual risk
  behaviors, 123

Racial differences
 abortion, 118
 HIV/AIDS, 119
 pregnancies, teenage, 117
 sexually transmitted diseases, 118
 sexual risk behaviors among
  adolescents, 115
Reducing the Risks, 127
Reinforcement, desirable behavior, 150–151
Religious beliefs, sexual risk behaviors
  and, 125
Research, recommendations for, 166
Risk
 alcohol abuse, high risk environments,
  49–50
 sexual risk behaviors, adolescents: see
  Sexual risk behaviors among
  adolescents
Runaways, sexual risk behaviors, 115, 122

SAMHSA: see Substance Abuse and
  Mental Health Services
  Administration (SAMHSA)
School-aged children
 antisocial behavior, interventions, 14–15
School-based curricula to prevent drug
  abuse, 94–97
 meta-analyses of effects, 96
 value of, 96–97

School-based interventions
 problem behavior, 153
 recommendations for, 164
 sexual risk behaviors, 127–129
 tobacco use, 67–68, 71, 75
 school policies, 68–69
Schools and Homes in Partnership (SHIP),
  104–105
School Transitional Environment Project
  (STEP), 15
Sexually transmitted diseases, 2, 118–119:
  see also HIV/AIDS
 urban youth, 123–124
Sexual risk behaviors among adolescents,
  113–143
 abortion, 118
 adjustment, parental influences, 125–126
 bartering sex, 115, 121
 behavioral dysregulation, 124
 clinics, school-linked, 129
 communication with parents, 126
 community-based programs, 129–130
 community-level interventions, 132–133
 consequences of sexual activity, 116–119
 delinquency and, 120
 dropouts, school, 120–121
 educational aspirations, 124–125
 ethnic differences, 115
 factors influencing, 124–127
  adjustment, parental influences, 125–
   126
  behavioral dysregulation, 124
  communication with parents, 126
  educational aspirations, 124–125
  intelligence, 124–125
  monitoring by parents, 126–127
  negative affectivity, 124
  neighborhood influence, 125
  parental influences, 125–127
  peer influence model, 125
  personality factors, 124
  religious beliefs, 125
 gay youth, 122, 130
 gender differences, 115
 high-risk subpopulations, 121–124
  gay youth, 122
  homeless youth, 122
  incarcerated youth, 122–123
  psychiatrically disturbed youth, 123
  runaways, 115, 122